Essentials of Plastic and
Reconstructive Surgery

D1101945

Essentials of Plastic and Reconstructive Surgery

with notes on clinical, nursing and general management

BRIAN MORGAN MB, FRCS

Consultant Plastic Surgeon, University College Hospital, London
and Mount Vernon Hospital, Northwood, Middlesex
and

MARGARET WRIGHT SRN, SCM

Formerly Nursing Officer, Mount Vernon Hospital,
Northwood, Middlesex

faber and faber
LONDON·BOSTON

First published in 1986
by Faber and Faber Limited
3 Queen Square, London WC1N 3AU
Photoset and printed by
Redwood Burn Limited, Trowbridge, Wiltshire

© B. Morgan and M. Wright 1986

British Library Cataloguing in Publication Data

Morgan, Brian

Essentials of plastic and reconstructive
surgery.
1. Surgery, Plastic
I. Title   II. Wright, Margaret
617'.95   RD118

ISBN 0–571–14501–9

Library of Congress Cataloging-in-Publication Data

Morgan, Brian
   Essentials of plastic and reconstructive surgery.

   1. Surgery, Plastic.   I. Wright, Margaret.   II. Title.
[DNLM: 1. Surgery, Plastic.   WO 600 M847e]
RD118.M67 1986   617'.95   86–11536
ISBN 0–571–13275–8 (pbk.)

Contents

Acknowledgements

Both authors warmly thank their many colleagues who have helped in the preparation of this book. In particular they thank Miss P. M. Walker MCSP, Miss S. Boardman MCSP, Miss A. Leveridge MAOT, Mrs M. Black LCST, Miss A. Ross CQSW and Mr C. D. Flood all of Mount Vernon Hospital, Northwood who have provided specific sections on treatment and management throughout the book. They also thank Professor J. W. T. Dickerson BSc, PhD, FIBiol for his help with the nutritional aspects.

Illustrations help to make a book come alive and for these they are immensely grateful to Mrs A. Besterman for the line drawings and Mr Blake for the photographs.

Finally, no manuscript can be presented to a publisher in an untyped state! Carol Brown and Caroline Barham typed and retyped uncomplainingly and are thanked most warmly for their endeavours.

Glossary

ABBÉ FLAP   A 'V'-shaped flap of skin, muscle and mucosa of the lower lip transferred to a deficiency of the upper lip, or vice versa

ABDOMINOPLASTY   (Apronectomy) Removal of excess of skin and fat from the abdomen

ALOPECIA   Deficiency of hair

ALVEOLUS   The socket of a tooth in the jaw bone and the part of the jaw bone where the socket lies

AMELOBLASTOMA   (Adamantinoma)   A rare tumour of the jaw which forms multilocular cysts. It does not metastasise

ANKYLOSIS   Joint movement restricted by fibrous tissue

APERT'S SYNDROME   An uncommon hereditary congenital abnormality which affects the shape of the skull and the facial bones. There are also hand abnormalities

AXIAL PATTERN (ARTERIAL) FLAP   A long mobile pedicle flap including a sizeable artery and vein running in an axial direction along the flap

BASAL CELL CARCINOMA (BCC) (Rodent ulcer)   A common form of skin cancer which never metastasises, but invades locally. Most frequently seen on the face and head

BLEPHAROPLASTY   The surgical correction of wrinkles and bags of the eyelids

BOUTONNIÈRE DEFORMITY   A deformity of the fingers seen in advanced rheumatoid arthritis of the hand and following injuries. The proximal interphalangeal joint 'button-holes' through the extensor tendon

BUCCAL   Relating to the cheek

CANTHUS   The angle at either end of the aperture between the eyelids

CAP SPLINTS   Shell-like metal dentures cast to fit the teeth exactly. They are cemented in place as part of the technique for fixing the jaws

CHEMICAL PEEL   Controlled burning of the skin, usually with phenol, to improve facial wrinkles or acne scarring

CHORDEE   A fibrous band where the urethra would normally be in the congenital deformity of hypospadias. It causes a downward curving of the penile shaft

COLUMELLA   The lower end of the nose separating the nostrils

COMPOSITE GRAFT   A free graft composed of skin and another tissue usually cartilage

CONTRACTION (of a wound)   Inward movement of the wound edges during the early stages of healing

CONTRACTURE (of a scar)   Shortening of a formed scar

CROUZON'S SYNDROME   Similar to Apert's syndrome but without the hand deformity

DECUBITUS ULCER   An ulcer formed from lying down, a pressure sore

DELTOPECTORAL FLAP   An axial pattern flap, q.v., from the chest and shoulder based medially

DENTIGEROUS (FOLLICULAR) CYST   A dental cyst containing a tooth

DERMABRASION   An operation for levelling off the pitted scars resulting from acne or smallpox

DERMATOME   A machine for cutting skin grafts which may be hand operated, driven by compressed air or electrically. The Paget drum dermatome is stuck to the skin to take an even thick split skin graft

DERMIS OR DERMOFAT GRAFTS   Shaved skin (maybe with fat) buried under the surface to repair defects of contour

DUPYTREN'S CONTRACTURE   Thickening and contracture of the palmar fascia of the hand causing the fingers to be pulled toward the palm

ECCHYMOSIS   Bruising

ECTROPION   Turning outwards of the upper or lower eyelids due to contracture or weak musculature

ELEPHANTIASIS   See lymphoedema

ENOPHTHALMOS   Sunken eye

ENTROPION A condition in which the edge of the eyelid is turned in toward the eyeball

EPISPADIAS A malformation of the penis where the urethral opening is on the upper side of the organ

EPITHELIOMA A squamous cell carcinoma of the skin

EPULIS Any tumour of the gum

ESCHAR The crust covering a burn. It consists of solidified exudate and dead tissue

EYELET WIRING Stainless steel wire loops fixed around the necks of the teeth to enable the jaws to be secured together

FLAP A mass of partly or completely detached tissue (skin, muscle, bone) transferred to a recipient bed and surviving from an intact arterial and venous circulation

FREE FLAP A mass of tissue separated completely from its donor area and transferred in one stage to a new site where the main artery and vein are anastomosed to suitable recipient vessels, usually using microvascular techniques. The blood flow is interrupted for a short time (1 or 2 hours)

GRAFT Skin or other tissue transferred from one part of the body to another without an intact vascular supply and nourished initially from the plasmatic circulation in the recipient bed. *Autograft* – from the same person; *heterograft* – from another human; *xenograft* – from an animal

GRANULATION TISSUE Repair tissue in a wound. It is formed by blood vessels and fibroblasts

GUNNING SPLINT Dentures without teeth made from metal or acrylic material to fit the gums firmly, used to help fix the jaw in patients without any teeth (edentulous)

GYNAECOMASTIA Overdevelopment of breast tissue in the male

HAEMANGIOMA A congenital vascular malformation

HAEMATOCRIT (Packed cell volume (PCV)) Estimation of the concentration of red cells in the blood. It is useful in monitoring the shock phase in burns

HELIX The outer margin of the ear

HIDRADENITIS A chronic inflammation of the sweat glands in certain areas of the body, usually the axillae and groins

HYPERHIDROSIS Excessive sweating

HYPERPLASIA Overdevelopment or grossly enlarged organ

HYPERTELORISM A rare deformity of the face where the forehead is broad and low and the orbits large and set widely apart

HYPOPLASIA Underdevelopment of an organ

HYPOSPADIAS A congenital condition where the male urethra opens somewhere along the length of the under surface of the penis instead of at the tip

INLAY MOULD A mould around which a skin graft is wrapped before inserting into a defect, for example on the inside of the mouth between the jaw and the cheek a buccal inlay is used

ISLAND FLAP A flap transferred on a subcutaneous vascular pedicle. It sometimes has a nerve supply as well, when for instance the surgeon wishes to transfer sensory skin from the ring finger to a denervated thumb

KELOID A pathological overgrowth of fibrous tissue in a scar

KERATOSIS Overgrowth of the horny layer of the skin. Can be pre-malignant

KIRSCHNER WIRE Wire laths of varying widths and lengths which have sharp ends and can be drilled through bone and used to stabilise fractures and joints

LEFORT FRACTURES OF THE MAXILLA A French surgeon, Le Fort, crushed the faces of cadavers and described 3 common fracture sites: I – low; II – middle; III – high

LENTIGO A freckle

LENTIGO MALIGNA (Hutchinson's freckle) A large freckle in old people which can develop into a malignant melanoma

LEUKOPLAKIA A flat white plaque on the mucosa of the mouth, sometimes predisposing to malignancy

LIPODYSTROPHY (1) Abnormal, usually symmetrical, collections of fat. (2) Faulty fat metabolism

LOBSTER CLAW HAND A congenital deformity of the hand which is shaped like a lobster's claw

LYMPHOEDEMA (Elephantiasis) A condition where the lymph produced in the limb is unable to drain away satisfactorily through the lymphatic channels and swelling of the limb results

MACROSTOMIA Too big a mouth

MALAR The cheek bone or zygoma

MALIGNANT MELANOMA A pigmented skin tumour

MALLET FINGER A deformity following an injury where the end of the finger (distal interphalangeal joint) cannot be straightened

MAMMOPLASTY, MAMMAPLASTY Surgery performed on the breast to increase or decrease its size and shape

MESH GRAFTS   Split skin grafts converted into a network and then expanded which enables them to cover a larger area or defect

MICROGNATHIA   Too small a lower jaw

MICROVASCULAR SURGERY   Vascular anastomosis carried out with the aid of an operating microscope

MIXED PAROTID TUMOUR (Pleomorphic adenoma)   A benign slow growing tumour of the parotid gland

MYOCUTANEOUS FLAP   A skin flap moved with the underlying muscle attached to provide a satisfactory blood supply. Common examples are the latissimus dorsi, pectoralis major, gluteus maximus, tensor fascia lata, gracilis and gastrocnemius myocutaneous flaps

NAEVUS   A birth mark

OBTURATOR   An appliance made to fill a hole or space

OCCLUSION   A meeting position of the upper and lower teeth

OMENTAL FLAP   A flap raised from the omentum and transferred from the abdominal cavity to close large skin defects. It can be moved on a long pedicle or 'free' with microvascular anastomosis of the artery and vein. It usually needs covering with a split skin graft

ORTHODONTICS   Prevention or correction of irregularities of the teeth, with appliances

OSTEOTOMY   A bone cut

PHARYNGOPLASTY   An operation on the pharynx designed to improve the nasopharyngeal sphincter closure usually in cleft palate patients

POLLICISATION   Reconstruction of a thumb by rotating a finger with its vessels and nerves and implanting it on the thumb metacarpal

PROGNATHISM   A condition where the mandible protrudes and the lower teeth override the upper teeth

RADICULAR CYST   A cyst occurring at the root of a tooth

RHINOPHYMA   A large red nose due to great thickening of the skin and sebaceous glands

RHINOPLASTY   Repair or reshaping of the nose

RHYTIDECTOMY (Face lift)   An operation to lessen the wrinkles and sagging skin of the face and neck by undermining the skin, pulling it tight and removing the excess

RODENT ULCER   See basal cell carcinoma

SAGITTAL SPLIT   A surgical procedure used to correct prognathism, *q.v.*, by splitting the ascending ramus of the mandible
and moving the jaw bone backwards

SCALD   An injury resulting from contact with moist heat

SEROMA   A collection of serous fluid (plasma-like) under a graft
or around an implant

SEQUESTRUM (pl. sequestra)   A section of dead bone

SILICONE RUBBER (trade name Silastic)   A man-made substance
used in the preparation of prostheses, implants, catheters and so
on, usually well tolerated by the body

SILVER SULPHADIAZINE   A preparation consisting of a silver
salt and a sulphonamide used as an antibacterial cream in the
treatment of burns. It is usually effective against *Pseudomonas
aeruginosa*

SPLIT SKIN GRAFT   A graft of skin taken through the dermis,
usually leaving sufficient dermis behind in the donor area for
the skin to regenerate from the hair follicles, sweat and sebaceous glands.

STENT   A term used to describe a mould. The name originates
from the firm that made a malleable dental material

SWAN NECK DEFORMITY   Hyperextension of the proximal
interphalangeal joints of the fingers, usually seen in advanced
rheumatoid arthritis affecting the hands, or after trauma

SYNDACTYLY   Webbing of the skin between the fingers or toes,
which can be either congenital or traumatic in its origin

THIERSCH GRAFT   A thin split graft named after the man who
first perfected it

TRISMUS   Difficulty in opening the jaws, usually due to muscle
spasm

TULLE GRAS   Petroleum jelly gauze. Marketed under various
names, for example Jelonet, Paranet

URETHROPLASTY   Reconstruction of the urethra

VOLAR   Pertaining to the palm of the hand or the sole of the foot

VOLKMANN'S ISCHAEMIC CONTRACTURE   Shrinkage and permanent scarring of the forearm muscles when they have been
without a blood supply for a length of time

WOLFE GRAFT   A full thickness skin graft used for small defects
particularly around the face. The common donor site which can
be closed directly is behind the ear; the graft is called a postauricular Wolfe graft – PAWG for short

Z-PLASTY A surgical procedure consisting of raising and transposing two interdigitating triangular flaps to form the overall shape of a 'Z'

ZYGOMA The cheek bone or malar

Introduction

The purpose of this book is to describe in simple terms the scope and practice of plastic surgery. It is intended as a guide for the student nurse, the trained nurse, and paramedical staff including dietitian, social worker, physiotherapist, occupational therapist and others, increasing their awareness of the important part they play as a member of a highly specialised team. Medical staff in other specialties, for instance general practice, often have little idea of the work of a plastic surgeon and it is hoped that they will find this monograph instructive and interesting.

The term plastic surgery was introduced by the Germans in the early part of the nineteenth century to describe the moulding of tissues. The use of plastic materials has nothing to do with the name and only rarely are synthetic materials employed. This is a surgery of technique and can be the practice and the treatment of many conditions. The work is largely reconstructive. The plastic surgeon deals with a number of congenital deformities, notably cleft lip and palate. He also deals with cases of trauma, particularly where there is skin loss and also facial fractures. Burns are usually managed by the plastic surgeon both in the acute stage and for the reconstruction of resultant deformities. Radical excision and reconstruction in cases of malignancy affecting the skin and also the head and neck are within his ambit. Aesthetic or cosmetic surgery improves the appearance of a person and corrects the ravages of ageing. Hand surgery is expanding to cover not only trauma involving the nerves and tendons, but also the treatment of rheumatoid arthritis. The increasing use of the operating microscope for joining fine vessels and nerves has made the replacement of limbs and digits a feasible and worthwhile pursuit. The design and application of free flaps and myocutaneous flaps makes the specialty an exciting one to be involved with at this time. The patients undergoing this intricate surgery need care which is specialised and of a high standard in order to complement the surgeon's skill and ensure the best possible results for the patient.

Records show that reconstructive surgery is an ancient art. In India about seven centuries BC operations were performed to reconstruct noses from skin flaps brought down from the forehead. It is said that amputation of the nose was used as a punishment for adultery and that a caste of potters performed the plastic surgery. The operation is still undertaken with modifications today and is known as the Indian method of rhinoplasty.

Tagliacozzi, an Italian surgeon of the sixteenth century, described an alternative method of reconstructing noses using a flap of skin from the upper arm. In his cases the damage was caused by duelling and also syphilis. From this time the knowledge of transfer of skin from one part of the body to another gradually increased, but it was in the nineteenth century, because of the introduction of anaesthesia and antisepsis, that reconstructive surgery really developed.

The First World War gave a great impetus to plastic surgery because of the great number of severe wounds caused by explosive shells. The work of Sir Harold Gillies was particularly noteworthy and he can justifiably be called 'the father of British plastic surgery'. Sir Harold Gillies inspired a number of other surgeons to specialise in plastic and reconstructive surgery, among whom were Sir Archibald McIndoe, Professor Kilner and Rainsford Mowlem. At the start of the Second World War a number of specialised units were set up and led by these men and others, and these regional units have expanded and multiplied to provide the plastic surgery service as it is today. The techniques devised for the accidents of war have been adapted and applied to the civilian and the domestic situation.

CHAPTER ONE

The Skin

FUNCTION

The skin acts as a protective covering to the deeper organs of the body. It is hard enough to withstand minor knocks and scratches and is readily replaced. The skin acts as a barrier against harmful micro-organisms, assisted by the sebum produced by the sebaceous glands. There are many harmful micro-organisms found on the skin but they only produce infection if the skin is broken. Great care must be taken to see that these organisms are not transferred to clean surgical wounds. Sensation such as pain, heat, cold and touch are felt by the nerve endings situated between the layers of the skin. Heat regulation is also an important factor. Heat is lost from the skin by radiation, convection and conduction and also by water evaporation associated with insensible perspiration. About 85 per cent of the heat produced by the body is lost by means of the skin in normal conditions. The skin is water repellent and enables it to act as the vapour barrier for the body. If large areas of the keratin layer are damaged, extensive fluid loss results and this can be seen in patients with large burns or de-gloving injuries. Vitamin D is formed by the skin when ergosterol found in the epidermis is exposed to ultraviolet light. This vitamin is necessary for the formation of bones and teeth.

STRUCTURE (Fig. 1/1)

The skin is composed of two layers; the outer layer known as the epidermis and the inner layer as the dermis. The epidermis consists of epithelial tissue and the dermis of fibrous connective tissue.

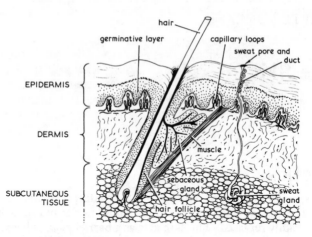

Fig. 1/1   The structure of the skin

The epidermis

The epidermis has several layers and varies in thickness in different areas of the body. It is the outer, horny or keratin layer that changes and the thickness is pronounced over the soles of the feet and the palms of the hands. The keratin layer is water repellent. The innermost layer of the epidermis, the basal layer, is constantly germinating producing new cells which move towards the surface, renewing the keratin layers as they rub off. Situated in the basal layers are special cells called melanocytes. These cells produce the pigment melanin, which affords protection against sunlight. A person's colour is determined by the amount of melanin produced by the skin and exposure to ultraviolet light increases the production.

Dermis

The dermis gives support and nutrition to the epidermis. It has two layers, the papillary and the reticular dermis. The predominant feature of the dermis is a fibre called collagen, and among the collagen are connective tissue cells of several types whose function is the destruction of the micro-organisms, removal of foreign bodies and repair.

The epidermal appendages, the hair follicles, the sebaceous glands and the sweat glands are found in the dermis. If the epidermis is removed by injury, it is the epithelial cells from these appendages that grow out to form a new covering. The sebaceous glands secrete a substance known as sebum and this, not only acts as a lubricant for the skin, but restricts the colonisation of the surface of the skin by certain bacteria, because of the fatty acids such as oleic acid which it contains.

There is a plexus of nerves deep in the dermis and fibres extend up from this to the basal layer of the epidermis so that if the basal layer of the epidermis is damaged in any way pain is felt. Sensation such as pressure, heat and cold are registered by corpuscles located in the dermis and the subcutaneous tissue; the sensation of touch comes from corpuscles just beneath the epidermis.

Blood supply

The largest skin blood vessels are found in tissues immediately under the dermis. They form a network, branches of which pass outwards to supply the skin. There is a mesh of vessels within the dermis and these vessels extend up to the basal layer of the epidermis, but the epidermis has no vessels of its own.

Lymph supply

The lymphatic vessels are also arranged in networks, and are very numerous in the skin. Their function is to reabsorb the rather larger molecules of protein and fluid from the tissues and return them to the circulation. Failure of this sytem, either as a result of disease or injury, allows fluid to collect in the tissue. This condition is known as *lymphoedema*.

WOUND HEALING

Wound healing takes place in one of two ways: *primary intention* or *secondary intention*. A clean surgical incision where the edges are held together heals by primary intention. A wound where the edges are wide heals by secondary intention.

The cause of the wound will play some part in the way healing will occur, but other factors such as blood supply, infection, and the presence of foreign bodies may well alter the healing process. A fine linear scar is the result of healing by primary intention whereas a broad scar which is less strong and poor in appearance results from healing by secondary intention.

Good nursing and high standards in dressing techniques can help to improve the healing by secondary intention.

Primary intention (Fig. 1/2)

The aim in all surgical incisions is for healing by primary intention. The healing process starts by the formation of a blood clot between the two cut edges of the wound. This acts as a seal. Epithelial cells grow out from the edges under the clot and push it to the surface where it is separated off as a scab. At the same time, deep in the wound, inflammatory cells, capillaries and fibroblasts are growing in. The fibroblasts form collagen fibres to provide strength to the repair. Healing in most cases will be established quickly, in about 4 to 5 days.

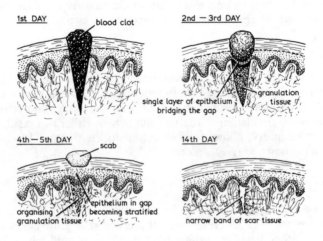

Fig. 1/2   Healing by primary intention

Strengthening of the wound will follow over the next 10 days but it will be several months for a soft supple scar to result.

At first the scar will be red and hard and then become white and soft some months later.

Secondary intention

In these instances the edges are wide apart and they may be separated by dead tissue, known as slough, which has to be removed, thus lengthening the healing process considerably.

The blood vessels and the fibroblasts grow in to form granulation tissue. There are many inflammatory cells stimulated by the presence of the slough and infection. The action of these cells and the chemicals from the granulation tissue slowly dispose of the slough and healing starts by epithelial cells moving in from the edge of the wound, but it is a slow process and the epithelium will cover only about 2mm every week. Wound contraction helps to bring the edges nearer. The end result of this process is a thin layer of epithelium which is very easily injured. Underlying this are collagen bundles forming a thick layer of fibrosis, which causes distortion as the fibres shorten and are re-modelled. This type of healing should be avoided and early removal of slough and covering the raw surface with a graft or flap is advisable. Careful surgery to preserve the blood supply and a high standard of nursing to reduce the infection are important.

The wound resulting from a partial thickness burn, or a split skin graft donor site is intermediate between the healing by primary and secondary intention. The epithelium is able to spread across the surface from one hair follicle, sebaceous gland or sweat gland to another, and as they are rarely situated more than 1mm apart, healing is usually complete at about 10 days.

Factors Influencing Wound Healing

Factors which influence wound healing may be divided into general (Table 1/1) and local (Table 1/2).

Table 1/1   General factors influencing wound healing

Factor	Effect
Vitamin C	This is necessary for the production of collagen. Most people will have sufficient in their diet but malnourished old people, those with debilitating disease or burns may need added ascorbic acid
Cortisone	Patients who are treated with cortisone heal less easily and the resulting scars tend to be weak
Protein	Patients with burns use protein as a source of calories, so this material is not so easily available for wound repair. Other conditions where the proteins are depleted may also have problems with wound healing
Anaemia	Wound healing is depressed in patients with a low haemoglobin
Uraemia, diabetes, jaundice, malignant disease	Delayed healing
Trace element, zinc	Deficiency in zinc is occasionally sufficient in old people to depress wound healing
Stress	In severely burned patients with very large wounds the stressful situation is sufficient to depress healing

Table 1/2   Local factors influencing wound healing

Factor	*Effect*
Ischaemia, infection	Patients with peripheral vascular disease heal poorly
Movement and repeated injuries	A healing wound should be rested and not continuously moved. Too frequent dressings can be harmful in disturbing the spreading epithelium. In a dirty wound however with much exudate, infection will delay healing so frequent cleansing is necessary
Foreign body	A laceration may contain a foreign body such as windscreen glass or stone from the wound and these may prevent the wound from healing. Surgically introduced material, for example a metal plate for bone fixation, if exposed in a wound will prevent healing. Dead tissue must be removed before wound will heal
Radiation	Tissues that have been irradiated over the 3 months previously will have a poor blood supply and heal badly
Site	Wounds of the hands and feet heal less rapidly than those on the face. It is prudent to leave sutures in place 12 to 14 days on the extremities whereas sutures in the face can be removed after 4 to 5 days

CHAPTER TWO

General Nursing Points

Plastic surgery is aimed at reconstruction and repair. Through the years there have been many advancements and new techniques devised. Modern science has brought new instruments and equipment, and techniques have been introduced which enable the surgeon to obtain better results and to extend his skills. However good the tools, results depend on many factors not least of which is teamwork between medical, nursing and paramedical staff; of these good nursing care is vital.

Patients undergoing plastic surgery often have to return to hospital many times before their care is complete. It is important that they find the surroundings congenial and that they feel confidence in the nursing staff caring for them. They will be anxious about many things, the operation, progress and the future: this anxiety will be increased at the thought of ultimate disfigurement or incapacity. Patients and their families and friends need constant support and reassurance, together with a deep understanding of their particular needs.

ADMISSION

Admission to hospital is the time when the patient feels at his most vulnerable, particularly if it is his first visit. A welcoming approach can do much to allay any fears and help to create a feeling of security and confidence. First impressions are important and the effect on the patient may influence his whole stay. Children in particular need careful handling for they are often very frightened; the nurse should be prepared to spend extra time to help them settle in. Courtesy and consideration should be extended to the parents who may be greatly disturbed by their child's admission, especially if it is as a result of an accident. A welcoming, compassionate attitude, with time to listen to their problems, will gain their co-operation and help to relieve their problems.

GENERAL CARE OF THE PATIENT

Diet

A nurse should remember that healing takes place only if the patient's general condition remains good; a well balanced diet is essential and the nurse should be aware of her responsibilities in ensuring that this is achieved. The advice of the dietitian should always be sought (see pp. 98, 118, 185). Diet is not always readily accepted by the patient, particularly if it is restricted in some way or not palatable. This is particularly true for patients who have had jaw surgery or those suffering from extensive burns. The nurse will require great patience and persuasive powers to gain the patient's co-operation.

Dressing techniques

Local care of the wound is of particular importance and a strict aseptic technique and high standard of cleanliness should be observed at all times.

Dressings should be performed in a special room set apart from the general ward:

(a) this minimises the incidence of cross-infection and
(b) affords the patient privacy during the dressing procedure.

This privacy can have the added advantage of giving the patient the opportunity to voice fears or ask questions he may not feel free to do in the open ward. Dressing change can be a lengthy performance and this time allows a good rapport between the patient and nurse to be established. For some dressings it may be possible for the patient to sit comfortably in a chair, but the nurse must ensure that the area to be dressed is well supported. For extensive or lengthy dressings the patient will be more comfortable lying on a trolley or bed and there will be less risk of the patient's fainting during the procedure.

REMOVAL OF SUTURES

Suture removal forms an important part of treatment and should be carried out with care. Patience and skill on the part of the nurse are essential; hurried or careless action during removal may well spoil the surgery. Suture material is fine and the loops to be cut small.

In all suture removal, four points should be observed:

1. Surgeon's instructions.
2. A good light, instruments, dressings and solutions ready.
3. Provision for the patient's comfort.
4. Provision for the nurse's comfort.

Good light: Excellent lighting is essential if removal is to be performed quickly, accurately and with the minimum of discomfort to the patient. It should be the nurse's first priority and she should not commence the procedure until she is satisfied she has the best possible illumination. A mobile light is an advantage.

Provision for the patient's comfort: The patient should be placed in a comfortable, relaxed position. The area from where sutures are to be removed should be amply supported and a second nurse should be available to assist the operator or to help reassure the patient. Two nurses are always required in the case of a child or a very nervous, apprehensive adult patient. It may be necessary to sedate children for some procedures – trimeprazine 2mg/kg body-weight given 1 hour before a change of dressing is usually effective.

Provision for the nurse's comfort: The nurse herself should be relaxed and comfortable. She should be able to move her fingers and wrists freely while supporting the elbows. Smooth steady movements with calm dexterity will give the patient confidence in the nurse's ability.

Method: Because of the nature of modern suturing material it is necessary to use fine instruments. Non-toothed McIndoe forceps and Iris scissors will suffice for most procedures but in some situations, on the face and particularly around the eyes, fine pointed forceps may be required to grip the suture ends. Disposable stitch cutters should *not* be used. The cutting end is difficult to introduce under the fine suture loops and there is a tendency to pull against the suture to cut which is painful for the patient. Good eyesight is essential to see the very fine suture loops.

If there is any crusting around the knot, the wound should be gently cleansed with a solution of hydrogen peroxide, sterile saline, or sterile water prior to removal in order to see the knot quite clearly and to avoid any pull on the wound edges when the suture is brought through the skin. The end of the knot is gripped firmly with the forceps and the point of the Iris scissors inserted under the loop at the side of the knot. The suture is cut close to the tie and gently pulled through the tissue by the knot.

The nurse should have a knowledge of the timing of suture removal in relation to the surgical techniques performed:

Face – 4 days.
Hands and feet – 12 days.
Other areas – 7 days.

She should be aware of what has been done and the type of dressing applied at operation, for example, a 'tie-over' dressing may have been used (see Chapter 3).

There is an increasing use of continuous subcuticular sutures: nylon or prolene zig-zags from edge to edge in the dermis of the wound. The ends are held with paper tape, beads and crushed metal clips or just tied together. To remove, one end is cut at the skin edge. The other is gripped with forceps and pulled firmly and steadily until the sutures slide out (Fig. 2/1). This suture can be left in a long time without leaving suture marks.

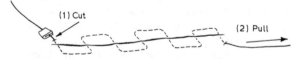

Fig. 2/1   Removal of a continuous subcuticular suture

Before commencing any dressing, particularly a first dressing after surgery, instructions should be checked, for instance 'remove dressing only', 'remove drain only', or 'remove alternative sutures'. It is important also to report accurately on the condition of the wound and to know what complications may occur and when to seek medical advice as to future treatment. Support of the wound may be necessary after suture removal particularly when it is performed early. The wound itself can be supported by applying sticky tape (Steristrip). In the case of a breast reduction operation bandage support will also be required.

GENERAL PRE-OPERATIVE CARE

Preparation before operation is similar to that for any general surgical procedures. Only in certain cases is it necessary to perform specific pre-operative care and these are described in the appropriate chapters. Scrupulous cleanliness is essential and the patient should have a shower or bath the evening before if the operation is scheduled for the morning, or the morning of surgery if the operation is planned for the afternoon. The surgeon may wish to mark the operative site after bathing prior to a breast reduction or flap construction such as a cross-leg flap. A good night's sleep is important and it is usual to prescribe a sedative to ensure this. Shaving of the operative site, if necessary, should be performed carefully and accurately. If possible, any specific postoperative positioning should be discussed with the patient so that he will understand the need for co-operation on return to the ward. The operation to be performed is explained to him clearly.

Most hospitals now have recovery wards close to the theatre where the patient first regains consciousness, and this means that the patient will awake to new faces. It is worth warning the patient of this, particularly in the case of the patient who has become very dependent on the ward nursing staff, and those who are noticeably anxious. Ideally, a recovery room nurse should visit the patient in the ward pre-operatively. It should be explained that the recovery ward is only a temporary stage and he will be returned to his own ward as soon as possible.

A parent, preferably the mother, should be encouraged to stay with the child after premedication and, if the anaesthetist is in agreement, accompany him to the anaesthetic room of the operating theatre. It is also helpful to let a child take a favourite toy or comforter along to hold until he is asleep. The parent should be in the ward to comfort the child immediately he returns, and then stay with him. (This will not apply in the recovery area.)

Many patients in plastic surgery units visit the operating theatre a number of times before their treatment is complete. The nurse should be aware that these frequent visits do not necessarily accustom the patient to the situation. In fact the opposite is true. In a number of cases, as treatment progresses, the patient's anxiety increases at the thought of further surgery and this is particularly true in the case of burns patients. A comforting, understanding attitude on the part of the nurse will help to calm the patient and encourage his co-operation.

CHAPTER THREE

Skin Replacement and Grafts

Skin loss occurs in injuries, full thickness burns, following removal of tumours, chronic ulcers and many other conditions. Where the area is small, direct closure by suture is possible but otherwise skin replacement is needed.

There are two techniques of skin replacement: (1) skin graft and (2) a flap. It is important to understand the difference:

A *skin graft* is a transplant of epidermal and dermal tissue which survives initially by nourishment from the bed on which it is laid.

A *skin flap* is composed of skin and subcutaneous tissues and this survives with an intact and functioning arterial and venous circulation (see Chapter 4).

SKIN GRAFT

Skin grafts vary in thickness. The skin may be 'split' either thinly (a Thiersch graft) or thickly. The whole thickness of the skin can be used as a 'full thickness graft' (Wolfe graft) (Fig. 3/1).

Split skin graft

Only part of the skin is removed in a split skin graft and the epidermis can regenerate from the epithelium lining the hair follicles, sweat and sebaceous glands left behind in the donor site, thus allowing spontaneous healing with little or no scarring. This type of graft may be taken from several areas of the body but the sites most commonly used are the inner aspect of the thigh and the inner aspect of the upper arm (Fig. 3/2). It may be applied to the

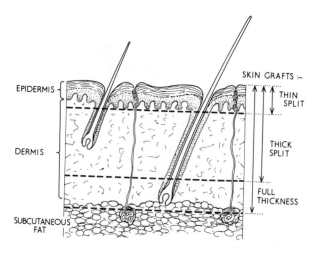

Fig. 3/1   The layers of the skin showing from where free skin grafts are taken

recipient area in strips or in large sheets, lightly sutured in position if necessary and left exposed or covered with a pressure dressing. A split skin graft will only take if the conditions are appropriate. There must be a good blood supply in the recipient area but because of the poor blood supply a skin graft will not take on bare cortical bone, over an open joint or tendon or where there has been irradiation. Much movement between the graft and the recipient area will prevent an adequate 'take'. A haematoma prevents the blood vessels growing through from the recipient bed and can prevent the graft surviving and infection, particularly *Haemolytic streptococcus*, can destroy a free skin graft.

The disadvantage of a split skin graft is that it tends to shrink or contract and if situated over a joint or mobile area can restrict movement. The thinner the graft the easier will be the 'take' but the more it will tend to contract. If mobility is likely to be a problem then a thick graft or flap is needed.

Full thickness skin graft (Wolfe graft)

This type of skin graft shows little tendency to contract. It stands

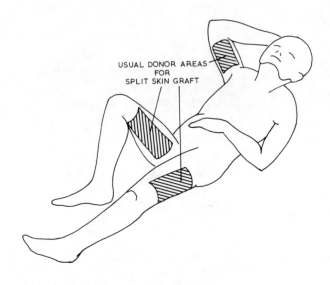

USUAL DONOR AREAS
FOR
SPLIT SKIN GRAFT

Fig. 3/2　The usual donor sites for split skin grafts

up well to pressure and has an appearance and texture nearer to normal skin than a split graft. Unfortunately, the donor area cannot heal spontaneously and must be closed by direct suture. This limits the size of the graft; nevertheless, it is very useful for small defects, particularly around the face where, if taken from a neighbouring area, the colour match is good. A common site for removal of a full thickness graft is from behind the ear and this is called a postauricular Wolfe graft (PAWG).

Taking a split skin graft

The first split skin grafts were taken with an old fashioned razor but Blair and Humby developed knives with rollers at the front of the blade so that the depth of graft could be easily altered. Special instruments used when taking a split skin graft are:

1. Braithwaite skin graft knife
2. Skin graft boards
3. Paget drum dermatome

4. Mechanical oscillating blade type dermatome
5. Skin mesher.

BRAITHWAITE'S SKIN GRAFT KNIFE

This instrument is a hand knife consisting of a slender disposable blade 24cm long fitted to a handle. It has a guide or roller in front of the blade, which adjusts the thickness of the graft. The donor site, usually the thigh, is prepared with antiseptic solution and towelled. Then the surface of the skin is smeared with sterile liquid paraffin or petroleum jelly and the assistant tightens the skin of the donor area by gripping the other side of the thigh firmly and flattens the donor area by pressing down with a graft board using his second hand. The graft knife is slid to and fro and gradually advanced and the split skin curls over the back of the knife as a sheet. When sufficient skin has been taken the graft is trimmed off with McIndoe scissors.

For ease of handling the skin is now spread on petroleum jelly gauze with the raw area uppermost. This skin spreading is carried out using non-toothed forceps and McIndoe scissors, being careful not to get grease on the raw surface of the skin. When this is complete the excess gauze is trimmed off around the edge. The raw surface of the graft is kept moist and covered with a saline swab until it is ready for application to the recipient area.

DERMATOME

The Paget dermatome is a half cylinder of metal, which is coated with a special adhesive. The drum is then stuck to the donor area of skin and the skin graft knife travels around the drum, cutting the graft at an accurate depth. The skin graft is then peeled from the drum. This technique allows a fairly thick graft of a large and even dimension to be taken from difficult donor areas such as the abdominal wall.

There are several types of mechanical dermatome which are operated either by compressed air or from the drive of a dental engine. The technique of taking the skin differs little from that used with a Braithwaite knife. The mechanical dermatome is particularly useful when large areas and strips of skin need to be taken rapidly in cases of severe burns.

Some surgeons stick adhesive tape to the skin before they take the graft and this avoids the necessity of spreading the skin later.

MESH GRAFT
If the skin defect is large and there is insufficient skin, it is possible to expand the skin by passing it through an instrument which cuts multiple slits and when traction is applied to the four corners of the graft, the graft expands and looks like a fish-net stocking. This has another advantage in that haematoma or exudate and infection can get out between the grafts and there is less likelihood of graft loss from this cause, but the final cosmetic result following the application of this graft is not as good as with a complete sheet.

Storage of skin grafts (Fig. 3/3)

Skin grafts can be stored in a refrigerator. The skin is spread on petroleum jelly gauze, rolled in a swab soaked in saline, then placed in a sterile container, with a few drops of normal saline, closed and sealed. The container is put in a domestic fridge and kept at just above freezing point. Skin stored in this way will keep up to three weeks and can be useful for later application in the ward or the operating theatre.

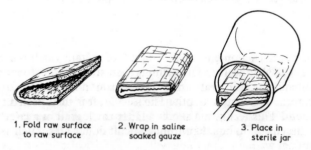

1. Fold raw surface to raw surface

2. Wrap in saline soaked gauze

3. Place in sterile jar

Fig. 3/3   Storage of skin grafts

The skin graft donor area is dressed with a layer of petroleum jelly gauze, followed by a layer of dry gauze dressing, a thick layer of cotton wool and kept in place with a firm crêpe bandage. The dressing should extend well beyond the edge of the donor area.

This dressing is left in place for 12 days, by which time the donor area should be fully healed.

An alternative technique is to use a clear plastic film, with a sticky surface, which is water vapour and oxygen permeable. (Opsite).

PREPARATION FOR SKIN GRAFTING

Three situations must be considered:

1. The defect of skin which is created in theatre during a clean surgical operation. Routine preparation of the surgical site, by shaving and cleansing in the ward prior to surgery, should be undertaken.

2. A recent clean wound produced by an injury or a burn. This area must be gently cleansed and shaved if possible and then protected with a closed dressing until the patient is transferred to the operating theatre.

3. A dressing or infected wound, ulcer or old burn. Extensive preparation of this area over many days is needed. Slough (dead tissue) is removed by gentle trimming and by the frequent application of a wet dressing. A suitable material to use is eusol (Edinburgh University solution of lime). This is effective only when wet and can be kept in a moist condition longer by mixing 1:1 with liquid paraffin. Dressing change once, twice or even three times a day will speed the cleansing of the wound and one can use a special apparatus to obtain continuous irrigation. Several proprietary de-sloughing agents are available of which Aserbine cream is probably the most popular. With this material, Aserbine solution should be used for cleaning the wound at dressings so that the pH is not greatly changed. A flat surface of bleeding red granulation tissue will take a skin graft; any dead slough remaining will prevent this process. An excess of granulation tissue is a disadvantage and can either be surgically trimmed, cauterised with a silver nitrate pencil, dressed with a hypertonic solution of saline or covered with Terracortril ointment. The surgeon usually removes the granulation tissue in theatre prior to grafting, to prevent excessive scar formation.

Immediate pre-operative preparation

The donor site is prepared by shaving, and if it is hair-bearing absolute cleanliness is ensured. The area around the recipient site is also shaved and cleansed. The surgeon may wish to keep the dressing in place with Elastoplast and the likely areas of fixation of this should be shaved. When the surgeon intends to expose the graft postoperatively, the patient should have this explained, and be prepared for a period of immobility to be necessary on his return to the ward.

NURSING CARE OF GRAFTS

Exposure method

A graft may be laid on the wound in theatre and left exposed. Alternatively, the skin defect may be dressed and the area left for 24 to 48 hours before the application of the skin graft, which is usually carried out in the ward by experienced nursing staff.

The success of the exposed graft depends very much on the care it receives during the first 3 or 4 days following the application. The area should be kept immobilised, and ingenuity on the part of the nurse will be needed to achieve this. Some form of splinting may be required or a particular position maintained. As the patient is immobile, careful watch should be kept for any signs of pressure in other parts of the body. The patient needs encouragement and moral support and should be kept in as comfortable a position as possible. The graft is inspected frequently. A gentle cleansing with some suitable solution such as normal saline or Savlon is performed. Collections of blood or serum under the graft must be eradicated and this is done by gently rolling out the fluid from under the edge of the graft, or, if it is centrally placed, by snipping through the graft and evacuating the fluid, again, by gently rolling. A dental roll or small ball of cotton wool may be used and turned with non-toothed forceps. The graft needs to be inspected every hour and haematomas evacuated as they form.

A DELAYED APPLICATION OF EXPOSED SKIN GRAFT IN THE WARD (Fig. 3/4)

The removal of the dressing that has been applied in the theatre can be difficult and painful for the patient and adequate analgesia must be given prior to the procedure. The dressing is gently lifted off using sterile saline to soften it where it is stuck. Some of the newer dressings, notably 'Release', come away quite easily without any pain. The area may bleed a little as the dressing is removed, but pressure for 2 minutes should stop this. The skin graft is removed from the refrigerator and appropriate pieces are taken from the sterile pot with sterile forceps. A graft not removed from the pot can be returned to the refrigerator, but once it has been taken out, it is inadvisable to return it. The graft is unrolled, spread on the wound, with the raw surface downwards; as it is laid out and stretched, the petroleum jelly gauze backing is taken off, as this only splints the skin graft and it is best to allow the graft to move with its bed.

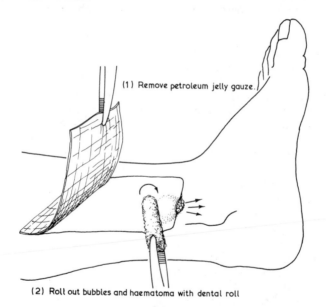

(1) Remove petroleum jelly gauze.

(2) Roll out bubbles and haematoma with dental roll

Fig. 3/4   Application of delayed skin graft in ward. Also showing how to evacuate fluid from beneath the graft using a dental roll

Any air bubbles, collections of serum or blood are gently squeezed out from the edge of the graft. It is surprising how quickly the graft becomes adherent to the bed but the edge of the graft may be secured to the surrounding skin with sticky paper tape (Steristrip) or cyanoacrylate glue (Super Glue).

PRESSURE DRESSING OF GRAFTS (Fig. 3/5)

In the operating theatre the graft is dressed as follows:
A layer of petroleum jelly gauze is placed directly over the graft; this and the graft are kept in place with a few interrupted sutures around the edge. Where there is a depression or hole, cotton wool soaked in flavine paraffin emulsion or normal saline is teased out and layered over the petroleum jelly gauze. Over this a layer of dry gauze dressing and cotton wool is applied and the whole held firmly in position with a pressure bandage or strong adhesive tape. This technique is particularly suitable for a limb.

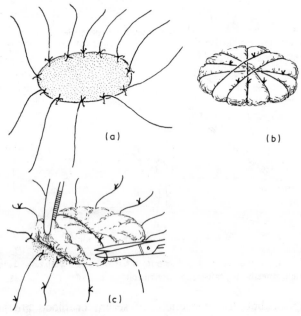

(a)

(b)

(c)

Fig. 3/5   Tie-over dressing

On the head, neck and trunk it is not possible to apply a pressure bandage and an alternative technique of tie-over dressings is used. Here the graft is sutured into position around the edge and one end of each suture left long. These ends are then tied over the flavine paraffin emulsion or saline soaked wool, pressing the graft firmly on to its bed. The dressing is then completed with gauze, cotton wool and a bandage or Elastoplast. Some surgeons prefer the use of polyethylene foam or wire wool. Grafts treated by pressure dressings are normally left undisturbed for 7 to 10 days.

First change of dressing

The patient is likely to be apprehensive; adequate explanation of the procedure must be given and the dressing carried out carefully and methodically in an unhurried manner. Calm dexterity by the nurse will promote confidence in the patient. The dressing is removed in the reverse order to which it was applied. First remove the outer bandage, the cotton wool and the gauze. The long ends of the sutures holding the flavine wool pad in position are carefully snipped and traced back to the edge of the graft (Fig. 3/5c). When all these have been divided the pressure pad can be removed. This may have become hard and adherent, however, and it will help to soak the pad with normal saline or sterile water. When it has become really moist it will peel away more easily, exposing the graft underneath. Any remaining sutures are then removed and the petroleum jelly gauze dressing last of all. The overlapping areas of graft beneath can be carefully cut away and the surrounding area gently cleansed. An alternative technique is to remove the sutures completely along one edge of the tie-over dressing, separate the petroleum jelly gauze from the surface of the graft at this point and then work around the edge of the dressing, removing the sutures and separating it from the graft bit by bit until it is completely free.

A further dressing may not be necessary if the graft has taken well, although it may be wise to apply a light protective dressing if there is danger of its being rubbed by clothing. A nurse should be able to determine the degree of take when removing a dressing for the first time and it is important to record this and report to the doctor. A graft which has taken well is recognised by its pink colour, which blanches on pressure, its slight translucency and its adherence to the underlying graft bed. In contrast, a graft which has not taken is pale and opaque and floats on its bed. There may be obvious pus or haematoma under the graft; the haematoma appears as dark red or black fluid or may even be solid. Part of the graft may have taken satisfactorily and another area not and it is important to note roughly the percentage of take, and the sites where the graft has not taken. Occasionally a graft which has taken well may have a loose film on the surface. This is called 'ghosting' and may trap the unwary into thinking that the graft has failed to take. It is due to the desquamation of the surface layers of the epithelium. Yet another appearance is of a seroma, where the whole graft may be lifted up by a straw-coloured or slightly bloodstained fluid. Surprisingly, the graft sometimes can survive over this fluid and repeated aspiration may result in adhesion of the graft to the bed and a resultant 'take', but this is not always so.

Care of donor area

Patients complain more of pain from the skin graft donor area than from the site of the graft application and analgesics such as paracetamol are needed regularly to ease the pain. The donor area will ooze for several days. The outer surface should be inspected frequently, particularly during the first 48 hours, and repacked over the top of the original dressing as necessary. It is advisable to leave the original dressing in place as in the early stages removal of this will cause bleeding and a lot of pain. The dressing is removed at 10 to 12 days. A very bulky dressing can make the wearing of clothes difficult and after 4 days some of the outer layers can be removed, making it less bulky, but the inner adherent layers must be left undisturbed. To assist early healing, it is wise to keep the limb non-weight-bearing for some days. A dressing on a thigh tends to slip down as the patient walks, causing pain and delay in healing.

The whole dressing is removed at 10 days; this procedure, which can be quite painful, is aided by allowing the patient to lie in a bath of warm water and gently soaking off the dressing. At this time the donor area should be healed and no further dressing will be necessary but protection against clothes' rubbing is advisable.

The patient is advised to bath and gently wash the donor area over the succeeding days and massage with hydrous ointment or lanolin. They should be reassured that sometimes small blisters can form on donor areas and that these should just be protected from further rubbing until they have healed. Donor areas itch a great deal and the patient should be warned not to scratch. The red discoloration of the donor area gradually fades over succeeding weeks and months and becomes a pale, just noticeable patch a year after the grafting procedure. Some individuals develop hypertrophic or keloid scars in the donor areas and will need to be fitted with an elastic garment (Jobst) or stocking (Tubigrip) (see p. 122).

The donor areas that are covered with the clear plastic film are not as painful as those covered with a conventional dressing and may be removed at 7 or 8 days. They do however collect serum or blood underneath the plastic film and if a large quantity of this is formed it is best to aspirate through the plastic film using a sterile syringe and needle. The aspiration hole can be sealed with a further piece of plastic film or gauze pad and bandage. As the plastic film is removed it may be seen that it is lifting the new epithelium away in which case it should be left in place for a few more days.

OTHER SKIN GRAFTS

Composite grafts

Under certain circumstances small areas of grafts can contain other tissues such as cartilage and are then called composite grafts. For example, a defect in the alar rim of the nose can be repaired with a composite graft of two layers of skin surrounding a little cartilage from the ear. There has to be a large edge to suture into the defect so that vessels can grow in quickly and easily for the graft to survive. This type of graft is usually left exposed and may cause some concern by appearing as a purplish-blue colour after 48 hours, but gradually this colour improves, becoming red and eventually pink. There may be blistering on the surface.

Homografts and xenografts

Grafting with the patient's own skin is called an *autograft*. Skin from other humans can be used but, unless it is tissue typed to match exactly the skin of the recipient, it will always be rejected after 3 weeks. It can however be useful in cases of extensive burns to provide a temporary cover while the donor areas from the first grafting procedure have time to recover. *Homografts*, as they are called, are obtained from relatives, other patients or from someone who has just died. These latter are cadaver grafts.

Grafts from animals are called *xenografts*. The skin of the pig has some similarity to that of humans and can be used for grafting. Freshly harvested pig skin will take, but is rejected after 3 weeks. Freeze dried or lyophelised pig skin is a non-viable product which can be kept on the shelf. It acts like a dressing only and will never 'take'.

Dermal grafts

If skin is buried in the body, it goes on growing and will tend to form cysts. If, however, the epidermis is shaved off and only the dermis buried then it will 'take' and yet not form cysts. This type of graft can be used to correct defects of contour, especially on the face. Fat can be left on the undersurface of the dermis and some of this will also survive as a dermo-fat graft. If much fat is transferred it will atrophy, and although the graft looks bulky to start, over a period of months it will lose up to two-thirds of its volume.

SURGICAL PROCEDURE
Full thickness skin is taken from the groin or buttock with or without underlying fat. First the epidermis is removed by shaving with a scalpel blade or a skin graft knife. The donor site is closed with sutures.

The skin at the site of the defect is undermined, and the dermis, flat or folded, is inserted, drawn into the defect with stitches pulled through the skin at a distance from the incision, and these stitches are tied over small bolsters of petroleum jelly gauze, cotton wool rolls or buttons. Pressure on the area is maintained to prevent exudate or haematoma and allow the graft to take satisfactorily.

NURSING CARE
Postoperatively the nurse must watch for any signs of haematoma or infection. The stitches tied over bolsters are removed on the 4th

day so as not to leave prominent suture marks. The donor area sutures are removed at 7 to 10 days.

Bone grafts

Bone may be transferred either as a free graft, without any vascular supply or as a vascularised graft, using miscrosurgical techniques. Two types of bone graft can be transferred: (1) cancellous bone (bone marrow) which can be curetted or spooned out of the ilium. This type of graft takes easily and is generally used as a type of cement around a fracture or occasionally to build up a contour; or (2) mixed cancellous and cortical bone. The cortical bone, although rigid, does not take easily and will tend to absorb over the months that follow the grafting operation. Cortical and cancellous bone grafts are used to replace bone that has been removed during surgical operation or lost as the result of a fracture. It is usually placed inter-positional, that is between two ends of relatively normal bone and under these circumstances will persist. Bone can also be used in an onlay graft to fill out defects on the face but there is a high rate of absorption of this type of graft. Grafts of cancellous and cortical bone are useful in reconstructing a nose which has collapsed as the result of injury, disease or previous surgery and at this site absorption is rare. The iliac crest or internal (medial) surface of the ilium is the commonest site for donating bone; rib bone can also be used and if periosteum is left behind new rib will form. The technique of vascularised bone graft is discussed in Chapter 4, page 61. The bone taken from the ilium leaves a large raw area of marrow which bleeds for a few days postoperatively and the surgeon will insert a drain. If it is a suction drain it will need a regular change of bottle; if it is a tube or corrugated drain it will need to be repacked. The drain is removed when the amount of fluid is negligible but it may be in situ for up to 5 days.

The hip wound is painful and the patient should be confined to bed for 5 days. During this time the pressure area should receive special care. Some surgeons use a local anaesthetic carefully introduced under sterile conditions into the bone graft donor site. The sutures are removed, from the recipient site at 7 days and from the iliac region at 10 days.

Note: If rib grafts are taken the nurse should be aware that there is a danger of pneumothorax developing and breathlessness or chest pain must be reported immediately to the doctor.

Cartilage grafts

A free graft of cartilage has the advantage that it does not reabsorb and can be put into a vascular area as long as it is well covered. It does have a tendency to warp and bend. Recently there has been an increased use of diced cartilage to fill up contour defects. This cartilage, when it has been cut into many tiny pieces, is introduced into a cavity using a modified syringe. For many years people have used cartilage as an alternative to bone to build up defects of the nose. The source of cartilage can be from the costal region, but small thin pieces can be removed from the concha of the ear.

NURSING-CARE
The patient may complain of pain in the ribs if costal cartilage is used. He should be encouraged to move as much as possible and sit out of bed 24 to 48 hours after the operation. Sutures are removed in 10 days. If large pieces of cartilages are taken from the chest, there is a danger of pneumothorax.

SKIN EXPANSION

A recent innovation is the technique of skin expansion. A silicone bag is placed in a pocket beneath the skin. It is attached by a tube to a reservoir and to a valve, which is also placed underneath the skin a little distance away. Once the wound is healed the bag is inflated gradually by injection of saline. This is accomplished by filling a 20cc syringe with saline, attaching a 23-gauge needle and injecting through the skin into the reservoir. Injection of 20–40cc at intervals of a few days or a week eventually fills the implant. At this juncture a second operation is performed where the bag is emptied and removed, together with the reservoir. It leaves redundant stretched skin which can be moved to an adjacent defect.

Many applications of this technique are being tried, the most common being in breast reconstruction after mastectomy where a large pocket can be fashioned prior to the insertion of the silicone gel prosthesis. It is also useful for stretching the scalp to close defects there or on the forehead.

CHAPTER FOUR

Flaps and Pedicles

A skin flap is composed of skin and subcutaneous tissue and this survives with an intact and functioning arterial and venous circulation. Most flaps retain an attachment to the body at all times so that the blood circulation can remain active throughout the entire transfer from donor site to defect. That part of the flap which remains attached is called the base or pedicle. Flaps, because they have their own blood supply, can be transferred to cover areas that are avascular, such as over bare cortical bone, an open joint, cartilage or bare tendon. Flap skin does not contract, so it is used to resurface areas over the front of joints and other sites where a split skin graft would shrink leaving a problem. The subcutaneous fat acts as a padding and is useful where skin has been lost over a prominent bony point. The texture of the skin in a flap is unaltered and so it will have a better appearance than a skin graft, particularly if it is transferred from an adjacent area to the defect, thus having a similar colour match.

The design, raising and transfer of the flap needs more skill than the use of a simple split skin graft. Surgical procedure is more time consuming and the postoperative nursing care is much more demanding.

Four types of flap are described – they differ in the way they receive their nutrition (Fig. 4/1):

1. Random pattern flap.
2. Axial pattern or aterial flap.
3. Myocutaneous flap.
4. Free flap.

The blood supply in the random pattern flap relies on the subdermal plexus of vessels and in order that the flap tissues should receive enough blood-flow the base or pedicle of the flap must be sufficiently wide. The length of the flap is limited by the width of the base and it is approximately a 1:1 ratio, thus a random pattern flap which has a width of 5cm should have a length of 5cm. If, however, a sizeable artery and vein are included in the pedicle of the flap and run axially in it, then the length of the flap comes much longer than the base and it is possible to slim the pedicle down to consist of only the vessels, leaving the flap as an island of skin. The main artery and vein of this type of flap can be divided, the flap transferred and, using microvascular techniques, joined to a suitable artery and vein in the recipient area. This is then known as a *free flap*. A multitude of small vessels pass from the surface of muscle to the overlying skin and large areas of skin can be transferred if they are supported by a transfer of the underlying muscle as well. Most muscles have an extremely good blood supply, often by only one or two large vessels. By cutting one or both ends of the muscle and swinging it on its main vascular pedicle, the overlying skin can be transferred in safety. This type of flap can also be used as a free transfer, dividing the main vessels to the muscles, and joining them up with suitable vessels in the recipient area.

Recent work has shown that the vascular plexus adjacent to the deep fascia can be harnessed to give added safety to a random pattern flap, and a fascio-cutaneous flap can be constructed considerably longer than a random pattern one.

RANDOM PATTERN FLAP

Local flaps

These are transferred from adjacent to the defect. They work well where the skin is lax and pliable, particularly around the face and neck and it is possible to close the donor site without leaving a secondary defect. If the donor site cannot be closed without tension, then this can be covered with a split skin graft.

Transposition flap (Fig. 4/2)

This is a square of skin transferred into a triangle figure.

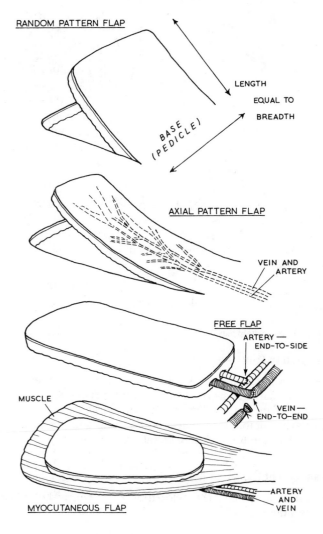

RANDOM PATTERN FLAP

LENGTH
EQUAL TO
BREADTH

BASE
(PEDICLE)

AXIAL PATTERN FLAP

VEIN AND
ARTERY

FREE FLAP

ARTERY —
END-TO-SIDE

VEIN —
END-TO-END

MUSCLE

ARTERY
AND
VEIN

MYOCUTANEOUS FLAP

Fig. 4/1   Types of flap

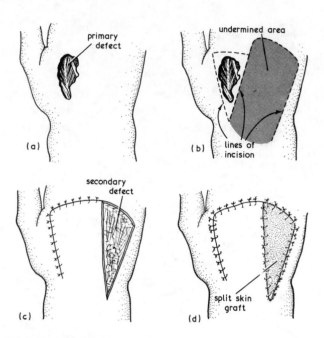

Fig. 4/2   Transposition flap

Rotation flap (Fig. 4/3)

Here half a circle of skin is rotated into a triangular defect. To advance the flap 2.5cm (1in) usually requires 20cm (8in) round the edge of the flap, so these flaps are usually fairly sizeable. They are particularly suitable for a defect on the scalp and cheek. Double rotation flaps are used to close sacral pressure ulcers.

Advancement flap (Fig. 4/4)

Skin cut as a 'V' and then closed as a 'Y' will advance tissue towards a defect.

Z-plasty (Fig. 4/5)

This is particularly useful for lengthening a contracted scar where

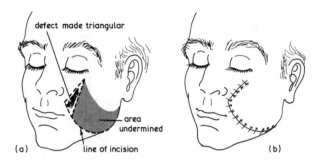

Fig. 4/3 Rotation flap

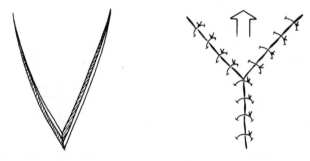

Fig. 4/4 'V' to 'Y' advancement flap

it has formed a web across the joint. Two triangular transposition flaps are raised on either side of the contracted scar which is removed. When the flaps are transposed, there is a lengthening effect and the scars have been transferred to a more advantageous position.

Distant flaps

Here the tissues are transferred from a donor area that is not adjacent to the defect. For instance, a defect of the skin on the arm or hand may be covered using a flap of skin from the abdomen

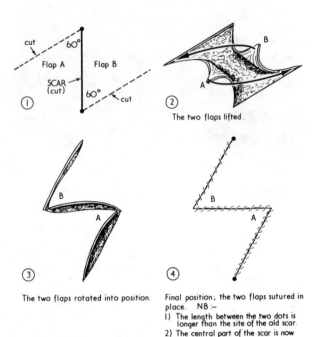

Fig. 4/5   Z-plasty

(Fig. 4/6). The tissue is raised on three sides, leaving the fourth side attached, rather like an envelope flap. The base of the flap is broader than its length. The flap is sutured into the position over the skin defect on the limb and then the limb has to be held close to the trunk, usually by strong strapping. The secondary defect on the abdomen is covered with a split skin graft or directly closed. The three edges attached to the limb heal and blood vessels grow into the flap. It takes between 2 and 3 weeks for the flap to become secure in this position. At this time the fourth side is divided from the trunk and sutured into place, completing the cover. Similarly a defect on the leg can be treated by raising a flap from the calf of the opposite leg, known as a cross-leg flap (Fig. 4/7). The two legs are held in position by plaster of Paris for 3 weeks before dividing the pedicle. There are other ingenious ways to keep the legs fixed

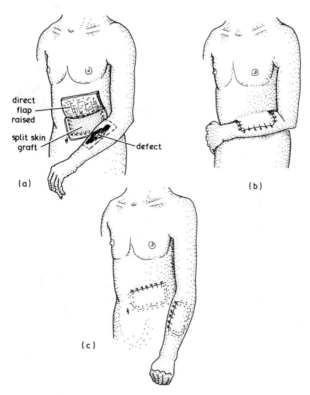

direct
flap
raised

split skin
graft

defect

(a)

(b)

(c)

Fig. 4/6   A distant flap: transferring skin from abdomen to the forearm

together, such as using a box with blocks of foam wedging the legs together or using a vacuum splint. Finger injuries can be covered with the flap from the adjoining fingers – these are known as cross-finger flaps (Fig. 4/8).

Tubed pedicle flap (Fig. 4/9)

There are times when the area for repair cannot be brought close enough to the donor site. Here the problem is solved by raising a tubed flap and using an intermediate carrying agent. The skin flap is raised along two sides and tubed. After 3 weeks one end is

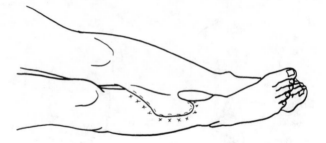

Fig. 4/7   Cross-leg flap

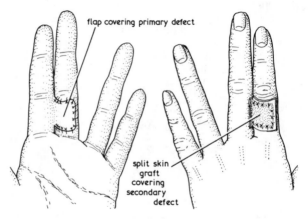

Fig. 4/8   Cross-finger flap

detached and transferred to the ulnar or radial border of the wrist. The wrist then becomes a carrying agent. When the tube has healed on the wrist at about 3 weeks, the second end is detached from the donor site and inserted at the upper or lower end of the defect. When this has healed and the blood supply into the tube has become adequate the wrist attachment is divided and inserted into the opposite end of the defect. Lastly, the tube is incised down the middle and spread. Each stage is separated by 3 weeks or more, so that this type of tissue transfer takes some several weeks to complete and is not commonly used now.

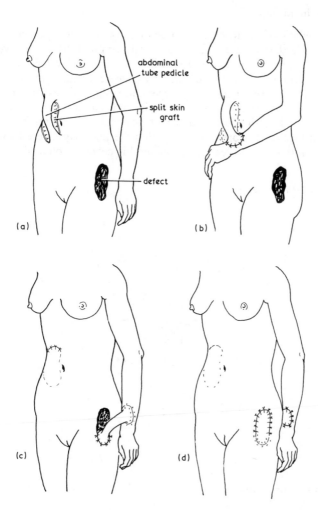

Fig. 4/9   Tubed pedicle flap being transferred from the abdomen

AXIAL PATTERN OR ATERIAL FLAPS

Forehead flap

The whole of the forehead can be lifted on a narrow pedicle from one side if it includes the superficial temporal artery and vein. This is a robust and very useful flap for resurfacing large defects within the oral cavity produced by excision of tumours; most of the patients requiring this surgery are old and because of the effects of arteriosclerosis, flaps in old patients are liable to necrosis, but the forehead flap is particularly robust. The disadvantage of the forehead flap is that the defect is covered with a split skin graft and leaves a considerable cosmetic blemish.

Groin flap (Fig. 4/10)

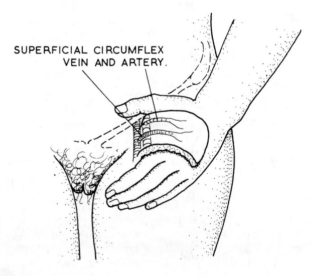

SUPERFICIAL CIRCUMFLEX
VEIN AND ARTERY.

Fig. 4/10   Groin flap

A long length of skin over the ilium can be raised if it includes the superficial circumflex iliac artery which springs from the femoral artery. This flap is particularly useful in providing skin cover for defects on the hand and forearm.

Deltopectoral flap (Fig. 4/11)

Skin over the front of the shoulder and chest can be raised on three arteries and veins which perforate through the chest wall, just lateral to the sternum. This flap finds use in reconstructing defects of the head and neck, particularly after cancer ablation.

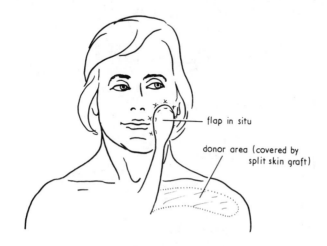

flap in situ

donor area (covered by split skin graft)

Fig. 4/11   A deltopectoral flap closing a defect in the cheek

MYOCUTANEOUS FLAPS (Fig. 4/12)

These are a recent addition to our armamentarium and new examples of these flaps are being described regularly. Some of the more common types are mentioned here.

Latissimus dorsi myocutaneous flap

A large area of skin over the back can be lifted with the underlying latissimus dorsi muscle. The muscle is detached from its wide origin from the back and swung on one of the main vessels that supply it from the axilla to a position on the front of the chest to fill

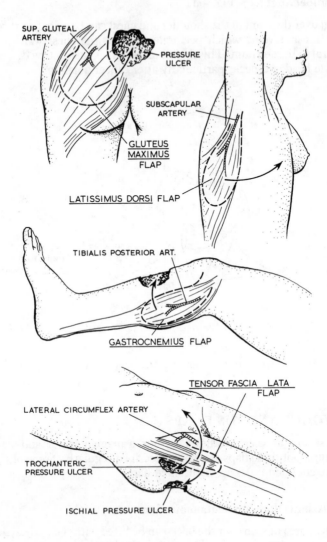

Fig. 4/12   Myocutaneous flaps

defects of the chest wall or breast, usually after ablation of breast cancer.

Pectoralis major myocutaneous flap (Fig. 4/13)

The skin over the front of the chest is raised with the pectoralis muscle and its blood supply which enters from just below the clavicle. The skin and the muscle are moved up to close defects on the head and neck commonly after cancer surgery.

Gastrocnemius flap

One or both heads of the gastrocnemius muscle, with the overlying skin, can be moved from the calf to cover defects on the shin or over the front of the knee.

Gluteus maximus myocutaneous flap

This flap is a robust flap, useful for closing sacral pressure ulcers.

Tensor fascia lata

This flap from the side of the thigh can be used to cover trochanteric pressure ulcers and defects of the groin and lower abdomen.

FREE FLAP

Though the compound microscope was invented as long ago as 1590 it was not until 1921 that it was used for surgery on animals. Very soon after, the ophthalmic surgeons began to make use of it, but it was not until 1970 that microvascular surgery began to be more widely used in plastic surgery. Many attempts were made to carry out micro-anastomosis and specially small instruments were designed for use in this technique. As well as its use to transfer flaps of skin, microsurgery can be used to replant amputated tissue such as fingers, toes or limbs. In the transfer of flaps it is a great advantage to be able to transfer tissue in a one-stage operation instead of four or five stages which take several months to complete. The flap consists of full thickness skin and subcutaneous tissue and is of the axial pattern type so that it contains a

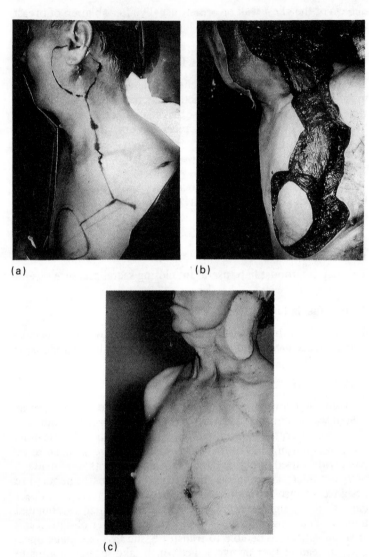

(a)

(b)

(c)

Fig. 4/13 Pectoralis major myocutaneous flap: (a) pre-operative marking; (b) raising the flap; (c) final result

sizeable artery and vein running up the centre of the flap. A good example of this is a groin flap, and the superficial circumflex iliac artery and vein are divided just as they come off the femoral artery and vein and sutured to a similarly sized vessel in the recipient area. The artery in the recipient area need not be divided completely as the flap artery can be joined at the side. A myocutaneous flap can be used in the same way. Probably the most useful flap of this nature is the latissimus dorsi myocutaneous flap where muscle and skin are transferred, anastomosing the main artery and vein to the latissimus dorsi muscle to a suitable artery and vein in the recipient area. Bone can be included in a free flap and these vascularised bone grafts are useful for repairing old compound fractures of the tibia and also for reconstructing the jaw bone. The ilium, with its blood supply from the deep circumflex iliac artery and vein is the most suitable site.

The surgeon needs to carry out a special pre-operative assessment, delineating the vessels, either with an arteriogram or with a flow meter (ultrasound.)

NURSING CARE OF FLAPS

Careful planning of the flap before surgery is essential. The surgeon will usually wish to measure and mark the flap and defect on the skin, and as he will not want the marks washed off the patient should be first bathed and clean. Although the part will need to be shaved, it is important that the surgeon *sees* the hairgrowth. A hairy flap transferred to a location within the oral cavity could cause problems. Planning of distant flaps is particularly important. It is necessary to ensure that the patient is able to maintain the position of attachment, with the minimum of effort and discomfort, remembering that this position will have to be maintained for three weeks. Before the operation the nurse should explain to the patient the position that he will have to maintain so that he will be more co-operative and understanding postoperatively. There are various problems associated with the nursing care of patients following flap procedures. The most common complication is damage to the circulation of the flap from tension, pressure or kinking.

The patient will return from theatre with fixation in place. It is the nurse's prime responsibility to see that this position is maintained at all times. On return to the ward careful handling and moving of the patient from trolley to bed is essential. Frequent observation of the flap, noting the colour and temperature should commence immediately. A normal flap will look pink and feel warm to the touch. A watch should be kept for kinking, undue tension bleeding or the development of a haematoma. Any change noted should be reported immediately. Failure to do so may result in the loss of time for remedial measures to the flap and possibly a complete loss of it. Undue handling or touching is undesirable, but any exposed suture line should be kept clean by gentle cleansing until the time for removal of the sutures.

An immobile patient is in danger of getting pressure ulcers and regular inspection and pressure area care is carried out. Patients with a cross-leg flap may be helped by having a Balkan beam over the bed with lines attaching the plaster fixation to counterweights. The patient can then lift more easily for essential toilet and sacral pressure area care.

Nursing care for free flaps

The first 48 hours are critical and require special nursing care. The flap must be observed for colour, warmth, bleeding or haematoma. New equipment is being developed to monitor the blood flow in the flap and the nurse will need to have instructions from the medical staff on how this is to be used and what changes in the records they should note and report. Half-hourly clinical observations of the patient should be carried out, recording the blood pressure, temperature, pulse and respiration. A 'special' nurse should be with the patient all the time for the first 48 hours. The operation is a lengthy one, lasting anything from 4 to 12 hours and this will have an effect on the patient's general condition. He will usually have been transfused large amounts of fluid during the procedure and the input and output of fluid postoperatively should be carefully recorded. Suction drains are commonly used and a nurse must check that a negative pressure is always present. The patient is on complete bed rest and particular attention must be paid to the pressure areas.

Flaps are best positioned elevated so that venous flow is aided by gravity, away from the flap. Suture removal from a flap follows the normal practice, as previously described. Sutures are removed from flaps on the face at 5 or 6 days unless the area has been irradiated, but for the limbs it is preferable to leave the sutures in place 12 to 14 days.

In flaps where a difficult position has to be maintained it is advisable to sedate the patient and give adequate analgesia particularly for the first 48 hours. Some surgeons will prescribe 6-hourly morphia on a regular basis, without the need for demand, for a 48-hour period.

Most flaps will be exposed so they can be observed. Intra-oral flaps however are often difficult to see and need a good light and spatula as a retractor. A pocket torch is usually sufficient but a large night torch or ophthalmoscope are not suitable.

Physiotherapy

This is of particular importance in the older patient. The aim of treatment is to relieve pain, maintain mobility and prevent joint stiffness. As the patient is often in an uncomfortable position, pain may occur due to spasm and joint stiffness. Relief may be given by the use of ice, massage and accessory movement. Heat, if given, should be by heat pads, which must not be placed in the vicinity of the flap or pedicle.

Postoperative nursing management

GENERAL OBSERVATIONS

Blood pressure: This must be taken and recorded at regular intervals. A hypotensive patient will have poor perfusion of the flap as he will have compensated by the vasoconstricting vessels in the skin.

Pulse/temperature: These must be taken and recorded regularly.

LOCAL OBSERVATIONS OF THE FLAP

Hourly observation of the appearance of the flap is necessary and the findings should be recorded.

Colour: Pink, white or blue.

Blistering or oedema: Mark the edges of discolouration and observe if it spreads.

Capilliary return: Light pressure blanches the skin which immediately becomes pink again as the pressure is removed. Delay in capilliary return means that there is a circulatory problem in the flap.

Swelling: This is due to oedema or haematoma.

Bleeding: Is this just from the suture line or is there haematoma under the flap?

Drainage: If suction drainage is being used, is it working and is there a vacuum?

Position: Is there kinking or tension of the flap? Pressure on a flap may come from part of the fixation or another part of the body and a tracheostomy tape has been known to kill a flap.

INSTRUMENTS
Check the blood-flow monitor and the skin temperature of the flap.

Action by nurse

If any of the problems just discussed are observed, action by the nurse and doctor must be prompt. Report any change in the flap to the surgeon and do not delay.

GENERAL
Keep the patient warm, a space blanket can be useful. A cold patient has a poor peripheral perfusion. Reassure the patient and give analgesics to patient if necessary.

LOCAL
Reposition the patient to correct kinking, pressure or tension. Remove a tight dressing bandage, or tracheostomy tape. Remember to position so that venous drainage is assisted by gravity.

REPOSITION FLAP
Cotton wool pads, gauze or blocks of foam can help to correct kinking. Bring the two ends of the flap together with Elastoplast to

prevent tension. Remove any constrictive dressing, bandage or tracheostomy tape.

Action by doctor

This may involve evacuation of haematoma, either by aspiration with a syringe and needle or by removing a suture and applying gentle pressure to the flap. If this fails the patient may need to be returned to theatre for the haematoma to be evacuated under a general anaesthetic; the nurse should think of this possibility before allowing oral food or fluid.

Hypotension will be corrected by giving intravenous fluid and blood. Increases in the tissue perfusion and prevention of red cell sludging is obtained by the administration of low molecular weight Dextran.

Some surgeons recommend local applications to the flap to reduce the oedema. Sodium or magnesium sulphate paste applied regularly every few hours is said by some to be of assistance. Inadequate venous drainage can kill a flap, and occasionally a flap with venous congestion can be saved by the application of leeches.

Kinking and tension of the flap can sometimes be relieved by the removal of one or two critical sutures. The raw area left may need to be covered with saline or petroleum jelly gauze dressing.

CHAPTER FIVE

Congenital Deformities

Congenital deformities are defects which are present at birth.

CLEFT LIP AND PALATE (Figs. 5/1, 5/2)

Clefts of the lip and palate occur as a result of breakdown in the normal lines of fusion during the early stages of fetal development. Clefts occur on one or other side of the lip; occasionally they occur on both sides. The cleft of the lip may extend back through the alveolus or gum to just behind the incisor teeth. The defect may not involve the full height of the lip – a *partial cleft lip*, or it may extend into the nose – a *complete cleft lip*. The cleft of the palate is situated in the mid-line and may involve the bone of the hard palate or the muscles and mucosa of the soft palate. Occasionally the palate may appear intact but there is no muscle union across the mid-line. This is known as a submucous cleft. Combined clefts of the lip and palate occur.

About a third of the deformities have a family history. Parents are not unnaturally often concerned as to whether a further child would be affected with the deformity and genetic counselling should be arranged. The appearance of a cleft lip in a newborn baby is quite a shock for mother and father and reassurance and explanation by the nursing staff, followed by an early consultation with a plastic surgeon, can do much to alleviate their concern.

A cleft lip can be a considerable cosmetic defect, particularly if a bilateral cleft lip, where the central segment unrestrained in growth sits almost on the tip of the nose. Surgical correction of the defect can produce a reasonable shape but the child will be left with a permanent scar. It is less easy to correct the deformity of the nose.

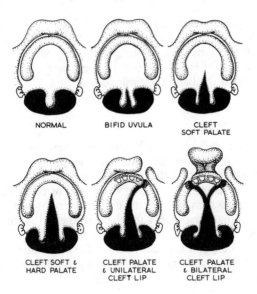

Fig. 5/1 Cleft palate

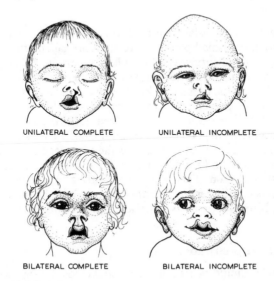

Fig. 5/2 Cleft lip

The cleft palate deformity interferes with function. It is necessary when sucking and speaking to close the mouth from the nose and to do this the muscular palate is lifted up to the back of the pharynx. Where there is a defect in the palate a seal cannot be obtained so that the baby is unable to suck.

Feeding

The inability to be able to suck is an immediate problem. Breast-feeding will not be possible, although the mother's milk can be expressed and then fed to the baby by bottle. Bottle feeding can be successful if a large hole is made in the end of the teat. Alternatively, a flange which fits into the defect can be obtained with the teat which is made especially for the purpose. If neither of these methods is successful then spoonfeeding is tried. An ordinary teaspoon will suffice and is usually successful but feeding is very laborious and time consuming and needs a great deal of patience by the mother.

Orthodontics

A baby with a cleft palate can be greatly assisted with feeding by the insertion of a small plate. Impressions are taken of the baby's mouth by a dental surgeon and the plate constructed. The plate is usually pressed up on to the palate by movement of the tongue and is secured by a tape to the cheek, or by two tapes around the back of the head, to prevent it from falling back and obstructing the airway. As well as helping with the feeding, this plate holds the alveolar segments in good position and, together with strapping of the external lip to pull it together, has the advantage of making the lip closure easier and producing a better alveolar (gum) arch and later tooth occlusion. This is called pre-surgical orthodontics.

The lip is usually repaired at three months and the palate at one year old. Neonatal repair is practised by some surgeons.

Pre-operative preparation

1. The baby should be free of coughs and colds, feeding well and gaining weight steadily.

2. The baby is better nursed in a cubicle with barrier nursing techniques in force.
3. Nose and throat swabs should be taken some days prior to the operation to eliminate the possibility of *Haemolytic streptococci* infections.
4. The haemoglobin should be 10g/dl.
5. Immediately prior to the operation the baby is bathed and the nostrils cleansed with water or saline.

The last feed is given four or five hours pre-operatively and should be a half-strength feed with added glucose.

SURGICAL REPAIR OF CLEFT LIP (Fig. 5/3)

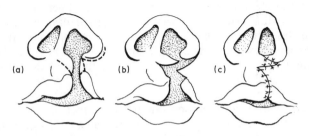

Fig. 5/3   Rotation advancement repair of cleft lip

There are several techniques, the most common being the rotation advancement method, as described by Millard. The medial side of the cleft is incised and rotated downwards to the level of the normal lip. The tissue on the lateral side of the lip is incised and advanced in to fill the defect created by the downward movement of the medial side. The cheek tissues are undermined and the nostril brought in to give a geometrical shape. The wound edges are carefully sutured without tension, using absorbable sutures in the mucosa and muscle, with very fine nylon interrupted sutures in the skin. It is unusual to use any dressing but the repaired lip can be protected with Steristrips, or a Logan's bow (a metal hoop taped across the lip). At the end of the operation it is inadvisable to use a normal airway as this would distort and press on the repaired lip. As an alternative technique for guarding the airway, a large suture is placed in the tongue. This stitch is left long and taped to the cheek where it can be pulled forward. This stitch is left in place until the baby is fully conscious.

Postoperative nursing

The baby is positioned on his side, with a very slight head-down tilt. Suction apparatus must be available at the bedside as there is a danger of blood running back into the pharynx, and the nurse should stay with the patient until complete consciousness returns. In order to prevent the baby's fingers reaching the mouth, the hands should be restrained and this can be done effectively by bandaging the arms to corrugated cardboard splints to prevent flexion of the elbows. The first feed of glucose water can be given about an hour after return to the ward and the baby is fully conscious. A half-strength milk feed may follow four hours later after which normal feeding can be resumed. If the mother has been breast-feeding up to the time of the operation, then she should be allowed to continue breast-feeding after. A contented baby is a quiet baby and there is less chance of bleeding or disruption of the sutures. Sedation should be avoided.

The lip sutures are kept clean and free from crusts by gentle cleansing with saline solution 4-hourly, commencing soon after the first feed. If a drink of cooled boiled water is given regularly after each milk feed, this will keep the mouth clean and further cleansing should be unnecessary. Lip sutures are removed four days after surgery. This is best done just after a meal, so that the baby is contented.

Occasionally light sedation is needed. It is important to have the baby firmly held so that the sutures can be removed without any pull on them which might cause them to cut through the edge of the wound and start bleeding. If necessary Steristrips are applied to support the wound after suture removal. The baby can be discharged from hospital the day following the suture removal.

CLEFT PALATE REPAIR (Fig. 5/4)

The object of surgery is to produce a long mobile palate, capable of lifting upwards and backwards and meeting the posterior pharyngeal wall, thereby closing off the nasal cavity. A leak of air will give a nasal tone to the voice and make certain consonants indistinct.

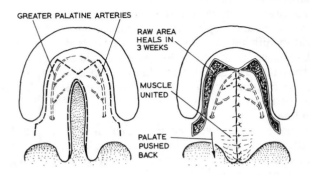

GREATER PALATINE ARTERIES

RAW AREA
HEALS IN
3 WEEKS

MUSCLE
UNITED

PALATE
PUSHED
BACK

Fig. 5/4   Wardil-Kilner cleft palate repair

The cleft palate is repaired at one year of age. The anterior palate in the region of the alveolus is best repaired at the same time as the lip, that is at three months. The technique most commonly used is the Wardil-Kilner operation where two mucoperiosteal flaps are raised on either side of the cleft, based on the greater palatine arteries. They are transposed medially to meet in the mid-line where they are sutured in three layers to close the defect. This leaves a gap at either side of the hard palate and this can be left open and heals within 14 days but sometimes it is filled with a Whitehead's varnish (Compound Iodoform Paint BPC) pack. The pack would need to be removed 1 week after surgery. The pack removal is best done by the surgeon under sedation or general anaesthetic in the operating theatre. The absorbable sutures of catgut or polyglycolic acid which have been used for the repair do not need to be removed.

Nursing care

Nursing care following this operation is similar to that given for the cleft lip. The child is admitted 48 hours prior to operation, so that swabs can be taken and an estimation made of the haemoglobin. Blood should be taken for grouping and the serum saved; some surgeons will also cross-match the blood of babies undergoing cleft palate repair.

Postoperatively the tongue stitch is left in place until the child is fully conscious. Closure of the cleft will have narrowed the airway to some extent and respiratory problems are possible. If there are respiratory difficulties, then humidified air is used or the baby can be nursed in an incubator. A close watch should be kept for oozing from the palate and the baby should be sat up as soon as he is fully conscious. Suction is carried out *only* if really necessary. Great care should be taken in directing the tip of the catheter so that the suture line is not damaged.

Cool boiled water given regularly after all feeds is sufficient to keep the mouth and suture line clean. Some surgeons advocate irrigation but it should be carried out very gently allowing only minimum pressure of fluid.

A feeding pattern can be established gradually in a similar way to that of a baby who has undergone surgery to the cleft lip. The baby is kept as quiet as possible. Long periods of crying are undesirable. The baby can be discharged from hospital 10 days from the operation.

Subsequent care

In most cases a good result is achieved by repair of the palate and a normal speech pattern will develop, but a scarred immobile palate results in a poor speech development; this can be improved by training the child to build up the weak pharyngeal muscles and to avoid the formation of bad habits. Because of the altered anatomy, these children are somewhat more susceptible to chronic ear infections, the 'glue' ear being a common accompaniment of the cleft palate deformity. The child may not hear properly. This affects the speech. On the slightest suspicion of hearing problems the child should be referred to the ear, nose and throat surgeon for investigations and treatment.

SPEECH THERAPY

As a member of the team caring for the child with cleft palate the speech therapist has several functions. First, she assesses the communication ability of the patient and provides remedial measures to improve speech and language. She may also be useful in liaising between the parents and the medical team and in assisting the

child to understand the surgical procedures that will be undertaken by surgeons and dentists.

In team discussion the therapist may be asked to answer the following queries:

1. Can the child learn to manage his present structures in such a
   way that good speech can be anticipated or should these structures be modified surgically or orthodontically?
2. If other treatment is to precede speech therapy, should the two
   forms of management be separate or can they overlap in time?
3. Are all the child's deviations in speech the result of the palatal
   cleft? How long a trial period of speech therapy should precede
   surgery in order to bring about desired improvement?
4. Is the child capable of acquiring sufficient linguistic skill to
   justify the long term surgical and dental treatment?
5. Will postponement of surgery create additional problems by
   giving the child opportunities to persist in faulty speech production?
6. Which is the greatest need of the child at present – more
   adequate dental structures, better velopharyngeal closure,
   improved appearance, or a combination of these?
7. How can the surgeon or dentist assess the child's speech to
   judge the effects of this management? What should he ask him
   to say other than sugar, father?
8. How does the child compare with the non-cleft child of the
   same age and development in speech and language?

Over the years the speech therapist's role has evolved from that
of clinician to that of diagnostician. In providing remedial assistance to the child the therapist's main concern is modification of
behaviour and therefore her relationship with the child is more
personal. This gives her more time to inform and influence the
child and his parents. The co-operation of the child and his family
is essential to the success of treatment and the therapist can assist
this by relaying and discussing the recommendations of the surgical team, encouraging the child to assist and co-operate in surgical
and dental procedures and to clarify terminology and provide
simple explanations for the 'glottal stop plosive, fricative and
affricable consonants', which litter assessments.

The speech development of the cleft palate child will deviate at
an early stage due to faulty neuromuscular patterns which are

established by the presence of abnormal structures. Speech is not established firmly in most cases until the latter end of the second year of life, although the actual sounds used in speech are acquired much earlier. Vowel sounds are often used expressively by the young babbling infant. At about 10 weeks the lips and tongue come into play and consonants make their appearance. Even a deaf child will babble. Gradually the vowels and consonants alter to resemble the sounds of language and self-imitation at this stage plays an important part. Syllables such as mum, mum and ma ma soon appear and the child makes good use of the soft palate, alternating nasal resonants and vowel sounds being an excellent exercise for opening and closing the pharyngeal sphincter. By the end of the fifth month the baby is responding to movement of mother's lips and will subconsciously imitate their action. If imitation were the prime factor, then, the consonants, p, b, and m, would develop first. K and g occur early, however, and s, z, sh, f, and u, develop later though sometimes not until there is adequate dentition or the alveolar arch has developed well. While experimenting with sounds the infant will gurgle and show general physical feats with arms and legs. This constant repetition is reproducing auditory images in the child's brain which in time become firmly established.

Parallel with speech and language development is a rapid growth in understanding. By the time the child is a year old he will understand far more than he is able to reproduce. Words at this stage are not differentiated but he is helped by intonation, facial expression and gesture. Once understanding is established progress is rapid and soon the child will produce a string of meaningless syllables with expressive intonation. As perception and muscular co-ordination increase a further stage is reached and the child will select and imitate a word just heard. The next important stage in development is the association of words with objects. A child will label an object and thus convey his meaning, for example, train, car.

The growth of language involves the ability to use words, thereby expressing thoughts. Vocabulary increases through experience, stimulus and intellectual development. The child progresses to phrases and ever lengthening sentences until fluent speech is attained.

There is a wide variation reported of phrases being used between 10 and 42 months, but it is known that the greatest increase in vocabulary occurs between 2½ and 3 years of age. This is a further argument against the postponement of surgery after the child's second year. In a survey of over 1500 children it was observed that two-thirds had defective articulation during the early stage of development. These defects occurred in non-cleft children. The speech therapist will try to make therapy effective by following as closely as possible the time development of the normal child, and using it as a guideline to treatment. The linguistic development is used to chart the point of break-down and subsequent build up of speech.

The child with mental retardation plus a congenital cleft palate will exhibit delayed language milestones and will probably have deficient articulation. Correlation between hearing loss and palatal clefts has been well demonstrated. Audiometry provides audiometric measures but further tests will be required. The hearing of children with middle ear infections is often inconsistent but any loss detected should be treated as soon as identified because of the close relationship between auditory ability and the discrimination necessary for the acquisition of adequate speech and language.

Evaluation of speech is a highly subjective process based on individual judgement and often more reliant on the human ear than the instruments of measurement. Even a group of speech therapists can disagree when listening to poor operative cleft palate patients. Instruments can supplement judgement, measurements of air flow, degree of capability, tongue position, palate pharyngeal closure and various aspects of phonation.

At the present time American speech pathologists as well as speech therapists practising in this country have found that the mechanical devices for assessing variability are not wholly satisfactory.

Overall findings relate to general information obtained from the following:

1. Malformation present at birth.
2. Surgical management.
3. Orthodontic management.
4. General physical management including paediatric care.
5. Family history.
6. Intellectual and emotional history.

7. Auditory activity.
8. Linguistic abilities.
9. Previous speech evaluation and general impressions.

The therapist assesses in detail the oral structures when examining the child before treatment commences. She looks at the hard palate, the soft palate for mobility and length; she notes if the tonsils are present and looks at the dental arch, its shape and position and finally she notes the mechanism of the velar sphincter when articulating ah or car. The appearance of the lips is noted: if there is a lack of symmetry, whether the child can round the lips as in pronouncing u, protrude the lips as in w, open the lips as in a smile and open and close the lips as in pronouncing m. She notes if there is any restriction in swallowing or chewing. Though she is not a dentist the therapist will also try to note if the arch appears proportional to the size of the head and face; which teeth are missing; the position of the teeth; which teeth are deciduous and whether the teeth are proportionate to the age of the child and if there are any signs of prognathism or retrognathism.

She will then define lingual mobility control. The range of mobility is important – up and down, forward and back, side to side. Does the back of the tongue elevate more than the front at rest? This can be beneficial in reducing slight nasal escape. Can the child swallow without tongue protrusion; can the tongue cope adequately with non-verbal activities such as licking the lips and eating? The state of the palatal structures is difficult for the therapist to observe but she will try to assess the length and mobility of the palate in conjunction with the pharynx to close the passage to the nasal cavities. A long but mobile palate cannot effect this nor can a short mobile palate. If the depth of the pharynx is great even a long mobile palate cannot effect adequate approximation of the structures. Ciné radiography or nasendoscopy enables the therapist to see the relationship between the soft palate and the posterior pharyngeal wall as well as the activities of the lateral pharyngeal walls as these also contribute towards pharyngeal closure. Direct observation of the pharyngeal structures is not within the province of the speech therapist; she is guided by audible cues as to laryngeal competence and she will test for nasal escape, whether it is excessive, moderate or pure nasal tone. An intelligent child from a caring background will often exhibit near normal speech though anatomically it should be far worse. Thus the criteria for speech assessment must be flexible.

Speech and resonance are assessed under the following headings:

1. Is there clear tone?
2. Is there increase in nasal resonance in conversation?
3. Is there further increase but still within nasal limits?
4. Is there nasal resonance but without nasal emission of air?
5. Is there nasal emission of air with marked nasal tone?

A mirror is used for testing, it will show clouding patches when nasal emission of air exists. All consonants are tested in initial, medial and final positions.

The Iowa Pressure Articulation Test was designed to evaluate the adequacy of velopharyngeal closure and includes consonant sounds shown to require the greatest amount of pressure through the mouth. As the test becomes harder with more consonant blends cleft palate speakers with inadequate sphincter make more errors. Certain sounds influence other connected speech and this is determined by dictated words, phrases and sentences. An attempt is made to observe the effect of nasal consonants on neighbouring sounds. Phrases not containing m, n are constructed and paired words such as men-bed, pad-pan, be-me, cup-come, hit-him, suit-soon.

It is important to test the sphincter competence on vowel sounds and sustained consonant sounds s/z f/v.

Positive consonant sounds p/b t/d k/g t/f d/z

Discrepancies between voiced and voiceless paired sounds are noted. Sounds in limited sequences are tested, what is the major direction of air stream or sound, for example, up, gay, easy, cat, spa, dress.

VC CV VCV CVC CCV CCVC

The use of sound in continuing sequence is tested, therefore obtaining a phonetic inventory of each patient. Listening is supplemented with observation that provides visual clues such as lip and tongue movement; construction of anterior nares, facial grimace and all attempts at velopharyngeal closures.

Treatment

1. Where paucity of language is evident and impedes communication, language rather than articulation training should be initiated.
2. A child with a severe hearing loss may not be able to profit from efforts to develop skills in communication until hearing has been improved by medical intervention or amplification.
3. A child wearing a dental appliance to correct a dental anomaly (should the appliance interfere with articulation), may be given only mimimal training or none at all.
4. A child with an unrepaired cleft or one who is to have additional surgery soon may profit from some general attention to sound discrimination or tongue control. This should make him more responsive to treatment following surgery.

A child who can produce good oral speech on command but lapses in contextual speech will need a different approach from the child who can control the sphincter but has formed the habit of substitution with glottal closure. Recommendations vary but guidelines can be given to parents should speech therapy be unavailable.

Most patients show a reduction in nasality postoperatively but where faulty habits persist a remedial programme is necessary. Programmes include ear training, exercises to increase the activity of the palate, yawning, air direction via humming games, blowing up of cheeks, using open vowels. The therapist uses a mirror and demonstrates to the patient and uses a multisensory approach both for work on deviant articulation and abnormal resonance. Short condensed courses of treatment are considered to be more beneficial than protracted courses of weekly visits, the aim being to have the child able to face the world at primary school with all his structures in good working order.

As the child becomes older other complications may occur. When the teeth erupt there may be irregularities for which special orthodontic treatment is recommended. Some deformity of the nose may persist which may cause distress or embarrassment to the patient as well as difficulty with breathing. This can be corrected by surgery. In the case of the cleft lip, scarring and shortening of the lip are seen in young adults and this can be improved by surgery.

Parents of these children are deeply concerned about their treatment and welfare, particularly if the baby is the first born. The nurse should remember that they require support and understanding at all times; the mother especially should be sympathetically encouraged in every way to take an active part in her baby's care and recovery. She should be taught feeding methods and, where they are applied, the care and application of dental plates. Any other particular points that may apply to her child should be carefully explained. When the child is at home both before and after operation, the health visitor can help and advise the mother, who should be encouraged to take advantage of this assistance. In some units parents are encouraged to meet other parents of children having similar deformity. They can then take part in free discussion and help each other greatly by exchange of ideas.

Secondary surgical management

Deformities of the alveolus and teeth occur and these can be dealt with by orthodontic treatment, although it is often not possible for the orthodontist to do extensive treatment until the permanent dentition has erupted. The child should be followed up regularly by the family dentist. Mother and child are encouraged to take great care of these teeth by regular cleaning and by the avoidance of sweets and Coca-Cola.

The child who has a satisfactory scar on her lip and a good shape of the nose with normal developing speech, needs no further surgery but is observed regularly until the age of 18. If the scar of the lip is unsatisfactory it can be adjusted just prior to school. A deficiency in the soft tissue of the upper lip associated with a bilateral cleft lip is corrected by an Abbé flap (Fig. 5/5). This consists of the transfer of a full thickness 'V' of the rather excessive lower lip to a deficiency in the upper lip. The flap remains attached to the lower lip by the labial artery and some surrounding mucosa for 2 weeks, when it is divided. The lips remain attached in the middle and so feeding can be difficult. Also, as these children have poor nasal airways, breathing may be affected but can simply be corrected by the placing of a large rubber tube between the lips on one or other side of the pedicle. The patient must be warned, prior to the operation, that he should refrain from trying to separate the lips until after the second operation. Speaking is not a particular problem. Following the operation the nurse should stay with the patient until he is fully conscious and aware of his surroundings. Careful suture line care and mouth washes or oral irrigation should commence soon after the operation and continue 4-hourly and after meals. A fluid diet will be necessary and this should be served attractively. It should be palatable and contain extra vitamins and be of high nutrient content.

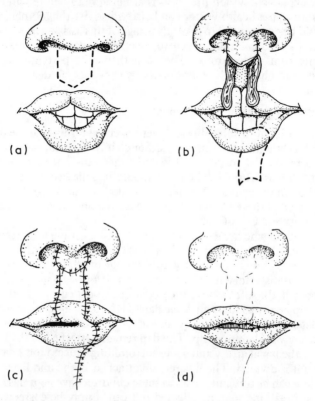

Fig. 5/5   Abbé Flap

Early suture removal is performed to avoid scarring. Division of the flap is performed under a light general anaesthetic at 14 days.

The deformity of the nose is usually more conspicuous and difficult to deal with than the lip scar. Small adjustments can be made while the child is growing but it is best to wait until growth is virtually complete at the age of 16 or 17 before a corrective rhinoplasty is carried out.

A cleft palate repair may be complicated by fistula formation or the palate may be short, scarred and immobile and this will produce marked nasal speech. Careful investigation is necessary. A speech therapist will spend several interviews assessing the problem. The palate is examined while functioning, through the front of the mouth, but a better assessment can be obtained by viewing the function of the palate through a telescope (nasendoscopy) passed through the nose (Fig. 5/6a). This investigation is carried out with the child sitting in a dental chair, awake and co-operative. The nose is anaesthetised with cocaine spray and the instrument passed. The appearance of the moving palate is displayed on a video monitor. Special radiographs of the palate can also be helpful.

PHARYNGEAL FLAP

It is possible to improve the closure of the soft palate by pharyngoplasty (Fig. 5/6b). There are several techniques in vogue but the two techniques most commonly used are:

(a) Superiorly based flap from the back of the pharynx inserted into the top of the soft palate (Fig. 5/6c).
(b) Two vertical and superiorly based pharyngeal flaps crossed over to make a muscular mound at the back of the pharynx.

Nursing care

Pre-operatively a throat swab is taken. The mouth and teeth are cleaned and the patient warned that he will have a very sore throat for a few days. Medical staff will arrange for blood to be cross-matched.

Postoperatively a watch should be kept for oozing or bleeding and for obstruction of the airway. Good oral hygiene should commence and continue at regular intervals. A fluid diet is necessary

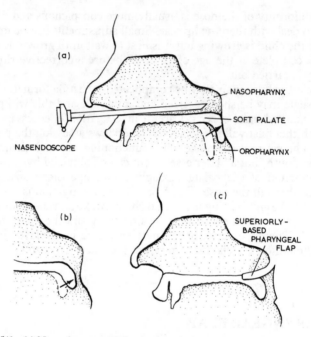

Fig. 5/6 (a) Nasendoscopy. (b) Incomplete closing of the soft palate.
(c) Pharyngoplasty using a superiorly based flap

for the first few days, later a soft diet may be tolerated. Both should have a high protein content and contain extra vitamins.

This is a painful operation and may be accompanied by stiffness of the back of the neck, probably due to interference with the vertebral fascia. Regular analgesia and a good deal of reassurance will be required.

In a proportion of cases of cleft lip and palate, there is a deficiency of growth of the maxilla. This may be due to the initial growth potential of the part but it could also be the effect of surgical intervention during the growth phase. Severe deformities can be improved or corrected with maxillary osteotomy or rapid expansion of the maxilla by orthodontic means followed by bone graft. These operations are carried out at the age of 16 or after.

HYPOSPADIAS (Fig. 5/7)

The male urethra instead of opening at the tip of the penis opens somewhere along the undersurface. The opening may be near the end (coronal hypospadias), or it may be situated beneath the shaft of the penis in the scrotal area or even as far back as the perineum. Associated with the condition is the downward curving of the penile shaft or chordee as it is called. This chordee is caused by a fibrous band formation where the urethra would normally be. This fibrous band is removed, thus straightening the penis and reconstructing the urethra with an opening at the tip of the glans, so that a penis is produced which is relatively normal in appearance and is able to pass urine freely and erect straight. Adults with hypospadias or repaired hypospadias are fertile.

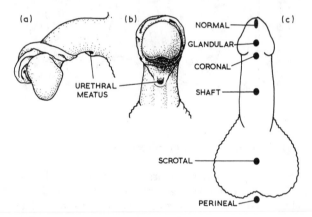

Fig. 5/7   Hypospadias

Surgical treatment (Fig. 5/8)

Many techniques have been and are used to correct this deformity. Where there are many operations to correct one deformity it is always a sign that no perfect treatment exists. The problem with hypospadias repair is the high incidence of fistulae and stricture following surgery. The Denis Browne technique is probably the most commonly used. It is planned in two stages. The first stage is

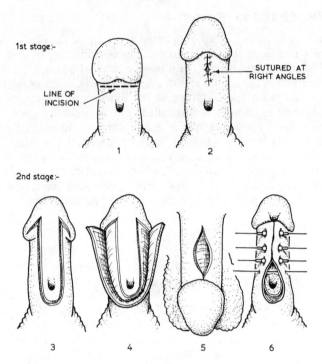

1st stage:-

LINE OF INCISION

SUTURED AT RIGHT ANGLES

1

2

2nd stage:-

3 4 5 6

Fig. 5/8   Denis Browne technique to correct hypospadias

carried out usually between the first and second birthdays and is to correct the chordee. Under a general anaesthetic the skin over the fibrous band is divided transversely, the band is removed and then the skin sewn up in a longitudinal direction. The second stage is carried out just prior to school. Many of these children have to sit down to pass their urine, or spray and wet their clothes, and it is best if this situation is corrected before it is noted by their peers.

To allow healing of the new urethra, the urine is diverted either by a perineal urethrostomy or by suprapubic drain. To form a perineal urethrostomy a catheter is introduced through the urethra; using this as a guide, an incision is made in the perineum and the catheter drawn out through this incision. Alternatively a self-retaining Foley catheter is introduced into the urethra in the perineum. The urethra is reconstructed by making two parallel incisions in the line of the urethra on the shaft of the penis. The skin to either side of these incisions on the shaft is mobilised up to the mid-line on the dorsum of the penis and then advanced to the ventral surface where it is sutured. In the original operation the sutures were held with beads and metal clips. If there is tension in the flap an incision is made in the dorsum of the penis. The wound is dressed and usually heals quite quickly. The buried strip of skin grows and forms a tube, which is the new urethra. The catheter is removed at 12 to 14 days. Skin grafts can be used to fashion the new urethra. Devine and Horton (1961) used a full thickness graft taken from the foreskin, which was then defatted and wrapped round a catheter of suitable size. The graft is sutured to the end of the urethra and brought out through the tip of the glans. To prevent contracture of both ends an oblique suture line is used with a small local flap at the glans. The foreskin is mobilised from the dorsum and brought round to cover the skin graft. The foreskin is an important source of skin for reconstruction in hypospadias and the parents of babies with this deformity must be warned not to allow circumcision. If circumcision has been performed the skin grafts can be taken from other areas but must be non-hair-bearing. At the end of both these operations a circumferential dressing is placed around the penis, which is then splinted to the anterior abdominal wall, using either plastic foam or dressings soaked in Whitehead's varnish (Compound Iodoform Paint BPC). This dressing is left in place for 7 days.

Nursing care

When the child is born the parents (father must be included) receive an explanation about the deformity and the necessity for leaving the dorsal hood or prepuce in place. When the child is admitted for reconstruction of the urethra a mid-stream specimen of urine is taken on the day of admission to ensure that no urinary infection is present. The nurse checks that the bladder is empty before the child is taken to the operating theatre. In all methods of correction an indwelling catheter will be inserted. It may be self-retaining or sutured around the orifice. The catheter and tubing must be secured with Elastoplast as well. It is a serious complication if the catheter comes out before its due time and usually necessitates the child's returning to theatre for a difficult reintroduction. Careful measuring and charting of the urinary output should commence immediately on return from theatre. Blockage of the catheter sometimes occurs and must be relieved urgently by irrigation. The child may experience some discomfort which can be relieved by suitable analgesia such as Panadol Elixir. Fluids should be given freely as soon as they can be tolerated to encourage the urinary output. It is advisable to splint the child's arms to restrain the hands in some way to avoid interference with the dressing. Regular inspection of the dressing and the exposed end of the penis is important and the dressing must be removed if there is congestion or excessive swelling of the end.

In some units the child commences saline baths 5 days after the operation. It is a help to put the child in a bath when the dressing is removed and the catheter taken out. At the time of catheter removal any retaining sutures are taken out. A Foley catheter is deflated and the catheter allowed to slip out while the child is in the bath.

Before the child is allowed home he should be observed passing urine of normal colour and adequate quantity.

HAEMANGIOMA

This is a congenital vascular deformity. There are three types.

Strawberry naevus

This appears as a small red dot shortly after birth and then enlarges quite rapidly to become a strawberry shape and colour. It can occur on any part of the body. They are often quite large and disfiguring and cause the parents great concern, but this kind of naevus undergoes spontaneous regression. The first sign of this is the appearance of a pale greyish area on the surface. Complete regression however may take five to six years and sometimes leaves a baggy area of pale skin behind. It is best to allow natural regression to take place and the parents will need a lot of explanation and reassurance. A few of these strawberry naevi, particularly if they are affecting vision, can be treated early by surgery or by using injections of sclerosant solution such as saturated saline. If an area of dry wrinkleless skin is left at the end of the resolution, this can be excised.

Port wine stain

The appearance is of a flat red or purplish haemangioma. It can occur anywhere on the body but is commonest on the face and neck. Unfortunately it does not resolve spontaneously and treatment is very difficult. The area can be excised and covered with skin grafts but this may result in unpleasant scarring. The laser beam is being used experimentally for treatment of this type of haemangioma and could be a useful method of treatment in the future. Cosmetic cover can do a lot to alleviate the patient's embarrassment, particularly in females. It is possible to cover the area using a selection of tones of cream make-up. Patients become very expert at application and complete the performance in a very short time. It is necessary for them to be taught the art of application and colour combination by a beautician and it can be relatively inexpensive if the creams can be supplied on a NHS prescription.

At one time tattooing of the dark red area with white titanium oxide and other pigments was carried out but this is less popular now. This type of deformity produces considerable emotional trauma when the child is young and if the parents are disturbed as the child becomes older and recognises the disfigurement, the emotional problems begin. It takes a great deal of persuasion and encouragement by others to help them overcome the stigma and seek advice and treatment available.

Cavernous haemangioma

These are bluish-coloured swellings, often rather deeper to the skin. They may occur in any part of the body and consist of large venous spaces full of blood. Occasionally thrombosis in them causes pain and swelling. Treatment is advised for cosmetic reasons and they can be injected with sclerosant fluids such as saturated saline, or excised.

A haemangioma that has developed an arteriovenous connection is a serious problem and one that needs urgent treatment. Fortunately this complication is rare. Investigation by arteriogram is carried out to find the feeding artery. Embolisation of the haemangioma followed within a matter of days by surgical excision is carried out. Simply tying off the feeding vessels may produce a temporary benefit but it is not long lasting.

PROMINENT EARS (Bat ears)

Prominent ears are common. They can cause great concern to their owners. Small boys receive unkind ridicule from their classmates and older people can find them a source of embarrassment. The condition may occur in families. Correction can be carried out from the age of six years onwards.

Surgical treatment

There are several methods of correction and every surgeon has his own variation. The commonest method is described. The operation is carried out under a general anaesthetic in children and sometimes under a local anaesthetic in adults. An oval-shaped piece of skin is excised from behind the ear. The cartilage is incised where the anti-helix fold is to be constructed. The skin is separated from the anterior surface and then the front of the cartilage scored to allow it to bend back in a smooth curve. This is a similar process to scoring along the dotted line of cardboard to enable it to bend and if this is done properly the cartilage will stay in its new position and the skin is closed behind. This is done with either continuous or interrupted suture. In children, surgeons try to use an absorbable suture to avoid taking stitches out of this rather difficult area. A bulky dressing using gauze cotton wool and a crêpe bandage is applied. The patient is allowed home after 48 hours but returns a week later for a check of the dressing position. The dressing is finally removed after 2 weeks.

Nursing care

Pre-operatively the hair should be washed. Some surgeons require it to be shaved around the ear. A margin of 2.5cm (1in) is necessary. Postoperatively the patient is discouraged from interfering with the bandages. Removal of the bandage is undesirable but if the patient complains of extreme discomfort, it should be loosened. The simplest way of doing this is to divide the bandage over the forehead, allowing a little relaxation and then reuniting the bandage with Elastoplast strapping. If the dressing becomes loose it must be reapplied immediately. Following removal of the final dressing, the patient is given a bandage to apply at night for the next six weeks in case the ears are bent forward while turning in sleep.

REFERENCE

Devine, C. J. and Horton, C. E. (1961). One-stage hypospadias repair. *Journal of Urology*, **85**, 166.

CHAPTER SIX

Trauma

The plastic surgeon deals with soft tissue trauma, maxillo-facial fractures and certain injuries of the limbs and hand – the maxillo-facial injuries with the help of the oral surgeons, and the limb injuries may well require the assistance of an orthopaedic surgeon. Much of the work results from road traffic accidents; soft tissue and bony injuries of the face are caused when the occupants of a car are thrown through the windscreen or strike the dashboard. These injuries are less frequent since the compulsory wearing of seat belts. Soft tissue injuries of other parts of the body may occur to pedestrians when they are struck by vehicles or may be caused by accidents in industry.

Motorcycle accidents cause injuries to the face and limbs. There is an increase in the number of compound fractures of the lower limbs with skin loss as a result of motorcycle accidents. This chapter concentrates on soft tissue and facial injuries. Hand trauma will be discussed in Chapter 8.

FACIAL LACERATIONS

Extensive and complicated lacerations are best dealt with under general anaesthesia; local anaesthesia is preferable for small wounds or in the presence of a head injury. Scrupulous cleaning of the damaged area is first carried out using an antiseptic detergent solution, taking care to remove all surface dirt and, if necessary, scrubbing any ingrained dirt that may be present in the wounds. This ingrained dirt, if not removed totally at the time of the operation, will result in the formation of permanent black tattoo marks in the skin at the site of the injury. These marks are difficult to remove at a later date and in some cases removal may be quite impossible. Once the area has been thoroughly cleaned, the wound is closed with careful suturing using fine suture material. The sutures on the face are removed in four to five days to avoid any marks.

Nursing care

Nursing care consists of 4-hourly suture line cleansing. The wound is swabbed gently using normal saline or an antiseptic solution of choice. Blood clots and crusts are removed as these cause moist wound edges, providing a medium for infection. Long, even strokes are used, alternately right to left and left to right across the suture line to avoid pressure on the wound. Any persistent clots are soaked with swabs dipped in a solution of hydrogen peroxide until they dissolve. They should not be rubbed virgorously. Lacerations near the eye are cleansed with saline only, as some of the detergent antiseptic preparations cause irritation to the conjunctiva. Sutures are removed at 4 days. It may be advisable to take out alternate sutures if there is doubt about the healing. If the surgeon has used an absorbable subcutaneous suture, then the skin sutures can all be removed together and at an earlier date.

FACIAL FRACTURES

The face can be divided into three areas (Fig. 6/1):

1. Lower third – mandible.
2. Middle third – maxilla, two zygomas, nasal and ethmoid bones.
3. Upper third – frontal bone.

Emergency treatment

In facial fractures there is a great danger of airway obstruction and the emergency treatment given at the time of the injury is important. Failure to understand this immediate danger and to deal with it effectively may well cause the death of a patient. The patient is often unconscious, has intra-oral bleeding and difficulty in controlling the movement of the tongue because of the swelling and

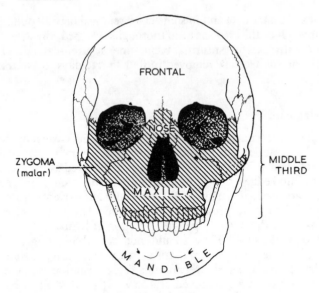

Fig. 6/1   Parts of the face for describing fractures

the instability of the lower jaw. Airway obstruction occurs. An adequate airway must be established immediately. The patient is turned on his side or prone (on his front) the tongue is pulled forward and the mouth cleaned of blood and loose teeth. The patient may then be moved from the scene of the accident. He should never be transported lying on his back, as the uncontrolled tongue falls back obstructing the airway.

Fracture treatment

The treatment of facial fractures follows the same principle as fractures elsewhere. The misplaced unstable fragments must be manipulated into the correct position and held firmly until union has taken place, usually about 4 weeks. Facial trauma may well occur in association with injuries elsewhere. The association of a head injury or chest injury, with a facial fracture, is particularly serious because of the airway problems. Serious limb or abdominal injuries could well take precedence to a treatment of facial injuries in the management of multiple trauma.

When there is displacement of a tooth-bearing fragment of bone, occlusion is disturbed. Occlusion is the relationship of the upper teeth to the lower teeth. The aim of treatment of these fractures is normal occlusion of the teeth when the mouth is closed.

As teeth are firmly fixed to the gum, they can be used as splints; when the teeth are correctly positioned the fractures will be reduced. There are several methods of fixing the teeth.

EYELET WIRING (Fig. 6/2)

Stainless steel wires with an eyelet at the centre are firmly fixed around the neck of the teeth on the upper and lower jaw so that they cannot be moved. Other wires are then passed between the eyelets on the upper and lower jaws and tightened until the teeth are fixed firmly in the correct occlusion. An alternative modern modification of this technique is to use an arch bar wired to the teeth, the arch bar on the upper teeth is wired to the similar bar on the lower teeth.

CAP SPLINTS (Fig. 6/3)

These are shell-like metal dentures moulded to the shape of the teeth and fixed to them with a very strong cement. They are made by taking an impression of the teeth from which plaster of Paris models are made and then on these models silver alloy splints are cast. Small metal hooks are attached to the splints so that the upper and lower jaws can be fixed together, either with wire or elastic bands. These splints have to be made in the dental laboratory and can take 24 hours to produce so that definitive fixation of a fracture is delayed one or two days.

For a patient with no teeth, it is possible to modify dentures and if dentures are not available, special Gunning splints can be made. These are similar to dentures but without teeth and they are made of metal or acrylic to fit the gum firmly. The dentures or the Gunning splints are fixed to the jaws with wires, through or round the bone and then the jaws can be held together by joining the splints.

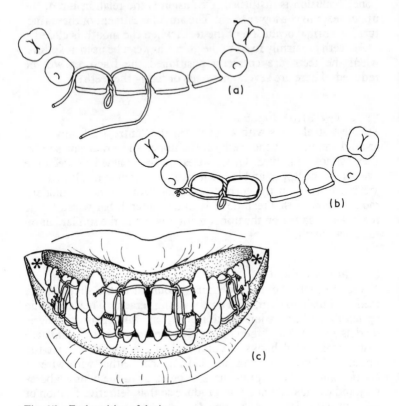

Fig. 6/2   Eyelet wiring of the jaws

INTEROSSEOUS WIRING (Fig. 6/4)
In this type of fixation the surgeon exposes the fracture by a surgical approach. Holes are drilled in the bones on both sides of the fracture and a figure of eight wire is inserted to hold it in a stable and reduced position.

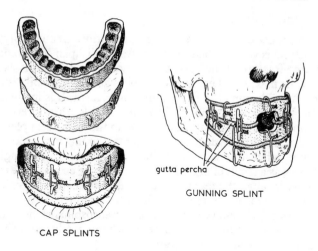

gutta percha

GUNNING SPLINT

CAP SPLINTS

Fig. 6/3   Cap splints and Gunning splint

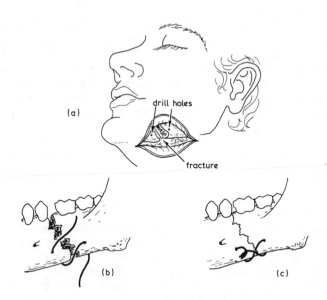

drill holes

(a)

fracture

(b)

(c)

Fig. 6/4   Interosseous wiring

Middle-third fracture

The appearance of the patient with a middle-third fracture is typical. The face is very swollen, with a flattened dishpan appearance, due to the fracture of the nasal bones and the backward displacement of the maxilla. There is a peri-orbital haematoma and distortion of the occlusion of the upper and lower teeth. It is important to look for clear fluid coming from the nostrils, this is cerebrospinal fluid (CSF) and indicates damage to the cribriform plate at the base of the skull with accompanying tear in the dura overlying the plate. When this is present there is a danger of meningitis developing as a result of organisms from the nose entering the cranial cavity through the tear in the dura. A combination of penicillin and a sulphonamide are prescribed for prophylaxis if a CSF leak is present. Excessive or prolonged cerebrospinal rhinorrhoea should be reported to a neurosurgeon, who may advise repair of the dural tear, using a fascial graft.

SURGICAL TREATMENT

This is usually carried out under general anaesthetic, although minor deformities can be dealt with without any anaesthetic, using gradual traction. First, the fractured bones are manipulated and positioned so the occlusion of the teeth is correct and second, the position is held by fixing the teeth together using eyelet wiring or cap splints (Figs. 6/2, 6/3). Sometimes it is necessary to stabilise the fractures further by fixation to the skull using external pins and rods, locking bars and universal joints. In the past a plaster of Paris headcap was used for fixation to the skull but now a metal halo or box frame is screwed into the skull. The jaw fixation remains for 5 to 6 weeks.

NURSING CARE

It may be some hours or even days before the facial fractures are fixed. During this time the nurse has to take great care to maintain the airway. An *unconscious patient* is nursed on his side and turned regularly. A *conscious patient* is kept sitting upright to reduce the swelling of the face. Regular oral hygiene is carried out, intravenous fluids given. The patient may be fed by mouth in some cases or alternatively a nasogastric tube is used.

Postoperatively the nurse's most important duty is to maintain the airway. The patient should be sat up in bed with a pillow support in an armchair position. Suction apparatus must always be available by the bedside, along with a tray containing wire cutters, screw driver and universal joint spanner for emergency release of the fixation should it be necessary.

In middle-third and multiple facial fractures swelling of the face may be severe and will increase postoperatively. It can be distressing to the patient when the eyelids are swollen and he is unable to see properly. If there is nasal swelling which, together with fixation, makes breathing difficult, he may be restless. Good positioning and suction will help, but firm handling and reassurance are vital.

ORAL HYGIENE

Once the patient has recovered from the anaesthetic, it is important to maintain good oral hygiene. If the jaws are fixed then this can be achieved by irrigation, using either a syringe or plastic squeeze bottle with a dental nozzle attached. There are many mouthwashes recommended. It is not the actual fluid that is important but the mechanical action of the fluid jet. A large quantity of fluid should be used. Particles of food very easily collect behind the teeth and between the sides of the mouth and the gums and they must be dislodged to avoid infection. Irrigation after every meal is necessary.

Technique: The nozzle of the appliance should be passed well back in the cheek to wash the debris forward and out of the mouth. A kidney dish is held under the patient's chin and he is encouraged to bend slightly forward and allow the fluid to flow from the mouth. The nozzle is directed along each side of the mouth in turn and then to the front. Irrigation continues until all the debris is cleared. If the jaws are wired the teeth can be gently cleaned using tooth paste and a soft brush or cotton wool wrapped round the end of a dental forceps. Care should be taken not to dislodge the wire. If metal splints are in place they too can be kept clean using a soft brush. It is important that the patients are taught to do their own oral hygiene while in hospital so that they can carry it out when they are discharged home with fixation still in place.

GENERAL NURSING

Fixation must be checked daily for stability and any loose wires or movements in joints reported immediately to the oral surgeon. If wires or joints are allowed to remain loose, redisplacement of the fracture(s) may result. If nasal splints are used they should be inspected for tightness and ulceration and cleaned 4-hourly. The holes in the skin through which external pins pass must be cleansed 4-hourly to prevent formation of crusts which may encourage infection. Surgical spirit should not be used as this enlarges the hole around the pin. A small piece of petroleum jelly gauze wrapped around the pin at its junction with the skin is an advantage. Metal rods used with dental splints may sometimes rest against the lips. They should be inspected for signs of pressure and if necessary a protective dressing wrapped around the rod. Swelling of the eyes is treated by bathing or irrigation with normal saline and the instilling of liquid paraffin drops every 4 hours. The patient will be unable to protrude his tongue because of the fixation and so cannot moisten his lips. To prevent them becoming dry and cracked, white petroleum jelly or lanolin must be applied. This will also help to prevent excoriation from the metal splints.

Patients who have the jaw fixed are often convinced that they are unable to speak because they cannot open their mouth. However, it is possible to speak without actually moving the jaws and a nurse can try this for herself by simply clenching her jaws and speaking through them. Patients will need persuasion that they can talk. Relatives are often alarmed until this is explained to them.

DIET

Following fractures of the mandible or maxilla, which do not require fixation, the patient can have a soft diet, which will not need chewing. It should be high in protein with added vitamins. If the jaws are fixed together then a liquid diet is given, which passes between and behind the teeth. A standard baby feeding cup with a lip and spout attached is an easy way to feed the patient. An alternative and rather older technique is to use a feeding cup with a spout to which is attached a piece of rubber tubing. The tubing can be passed along the inside of the cheek to the space at the back of the teeth and the feeder tipped to allow the diet into the patient's mouth.

Some patients find it difficult to accept a totally fluid diet, particularly as it is often not very palatable. The diet should be kept high in protein, vitamins and calories and supplemented with extra milk and eggs. The nurse will need to use her ingenuity to persuade the patient to tolerate this diet and if it is made to look attractive, this helps considerably. The dietitian should see the patient and his family before discharge and provide a diet sheet. A liquidiser is helpful both in the ward and at home, as a normal meal can be reduced to a form which is acceptable. Baby foods are useful.

Fractures of the mandible (Fig. 6/5)

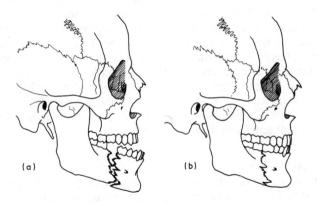

Fig. 6/5   Fracture of the mandible: (a) displaced fragment; (b) after reduction, checking the occlusion of the teeth

Fractures of the mandible may present on their own or in conjunction with other facial fractures. The fragments may be displaced (Fig. 6/5a) or undisplaced. Most fractures are compound, with lacerations either externally or intra-orally. The patient will have localised pain, particularly on opening the mouth. Movement of the jaw is difficult and there is swelling.

TREATMENT
The fragments are manipulated into the correct position and

checked by observing the occlusion of the teeth (Fig. 6/5b). The bones are held in position by fixation to the nearest stable bone, that is usually the maxilla (upper jaw). Fixation is by eyelet wiring, cap splints or modification of the patient's own dentures or Gunning splints (Fig. 6/3).

In some cases interosseous wiring is used, or, as an alternative, a small metal plate can be fixed across the fracture screwing it to either side and stabilising it. Fractures of the condyles are often left unfixed or intermaxillary fixation for a short period of time is used.

NURSING CARE

The patient should be nursed sitting up comfortably in bed immediately on return to consciousness. Suction apparatus should be available at the bedside, and if the jaws are fixed the care described on page 97 should be given. If no intermaxillary fixation is used then oral hygiene with mouthwashes, cleansing of the teeth with a soft brush and dental cream will be adequate. Extra fluids are encouraged. A liquid diet is not necessary; a soft diet which requires no chewing will be satisfactory. These patients are usually discharged quickly but before they leave the ward they should be taught oral toilet and dietary requirement.

PHYSIOTHERAPY

As most of these patients present as an emergency the physiotherapist does not see them until after surgery when the jaws are splinted or wired and the nose packed if involved in the injury.

Breathing exercises are carried out as the patient may have a considerable amount of blood in the mouth and back of the throat which could lead to chest complications. If the teeth are wired together, difficulty may be experienced in expectorating. Suction is carried out through the gap in the interdental wiring. Packing of the nose, if present, will exclude nasal suction.

When the splints are removed, if trismus is present short wave diathermy to the temporomandibular joint may be given.

FRACTURED NOSE (Fig. 6/6)

This is a common injury which usually results from a direct blow to the nose. Fractures may occur on their own or they may be part of other injuries. If the blow is from the side there will be deviation of the nose from the mid-line. If the blow is from the front there will be depression of the profile and splaying of the nasal bones. There is often damage and distortion of the septum and if uncorrected this obstructs the nasal airway, an unpleasant sequelae of this injury.

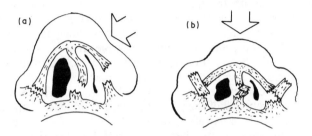

Fig. 6/6   Nasal fractures: (a) from a sideways blow; (b) from a frontal blow

Swelling of the nose is often marked and it may be necessary to delay correction of the deformity for some days to allow it to abate. Treatment *must* be completed by 3 weeks post-injury, however, as after this time fractures become sticky and are difficult to move. The aim of treatment is to restore the appearance and reposition the septum to avoid obstruction of the airway.

Surgical procedure

Under a general anaesthetic using endotracheal anaesthesia, the nasal bones and the septum are manipulated into position. This position is maintained by the application of a plaster of Paris splint and small petroleum jelly gauze packs are inserted into the nostrils. If comminution is gross and the nasal bones badly displaced, it may be necessary to put in a through-and-through wire suture tied over metal plates on either sides of the bridge.

Nursing care

Postoperatively, the patient is sat up as soon as possible as there may be bleeding from the nostrils and this position keeps the bruising and swelling around the eyes to a minimum. Cold compresses are applied to the eyes to reduce the swelling. If lead plates are fixed they will need 4-hourly attention to keep them clean and inspection for undue pressure or ulceration. After 48 hours the nasal packs are removed. The patient is positioned sitting up in bed, with his head firmly against the pillow. A kidney dish is placed underneath the nose and, after loosening of the external part of the gauze pack, the pack is removed with a Tilley's forceps. There is often mucus on the pack and this allows it to slip out without difficulty, but sometimes brisk bleeding occurs and the patient should be sat forward so that he does not swallow the blood; within a few minutes the bleeding will stop and after an hour the patient can be allowed home. The patient returns to hospital for the removal of the plaster of Paris splint as an outpatient on the 10th or 14th day after surgery. The Elastoplast is loosened using plaster remover or ether, being careful to keep the patient's eyes closed. The splint lifts off easily and after further cleansing the patient is allowed home.

Patients should be instructed to wash the skin normally but to be careful not to knock the nose. Make-up may be applied. The discomfort of a blocked or discharging nose can be relieved if the patient takes regular saline sniffs. He is advised to have a bowl of tepid tap water, to which half a tablespoon of kitchen salt is added, and with his head forward to dip his nose into the bowl and sniff up until the salt passes down the back of the pharynx. Although not very pleasant to do, this relieves the discomfort of obstruction.

FRACTURED ZYGOMA

This fracture is caused by a direct blow to the cheek. There is local swelling, anaesthesia of the upper lip caused by compression of the infra-orbital nerve, and double vision.

Surgical procedure

A malar elevator rather like a tyre lever is inserted through an incision in the temporal region, passed under the zygoma, which is lifted into the correct position. Most fractures remain stable but occasionally the fragments need to be fixed in place by inter-osseous wiring or by external pins to a stable skull or forehead.

Nursing care

The patient must not lie on the fractured cheek after it has been reduced, as it can be redisplaced by pressure. The surgeon will mark the cheek to remind one to avoid pressure. Four-hourly suture line care and mouth care should be established and continued as long as the patient remains in hospital. A soft diet is advisable and the patient should continue this on discharge. If pin fixation is used, 4-hourly care of the pin holes will be necessary.

FRACTURE OF THE ORBITAL FLOOR

A blow-out fracture of the orbital floor is caused by a direct injury to the eyeball with small objects such as a golf ball or squash ball, or even an elbow. There is a peri-orbital haematoma and double vision.

A comminuted fracture of the zygomatic bone may also be associated with gross disruption of the orbital floor. There is a tendency for the orbital contents to drop down into the antrum. At surgery the contents are elevated and a silicone plastic plate is inserted to make a new orbital floor and keep the globe of the eye in the correct position. Antral packs or balloons used to be used to push the orbital floor up from below and keep it in position until it consolidated at about 3 weeks from the time of the injury.

SKIN LOSS

The plastic surgeon deals with skin loss from trauma on the trunk and limbs. This may be a trivial injury or a major problem with extensive loss of skin such as in a de-gloving injury or associated with fractures.

A common trivial injury is for middle-aged or elderly women to knock the front of their shins on a household object, such as a coal bucket, lifting a 'V'-shaped flap of skin which is non-vital. It is best to treat this straight away by excising the flap and putting on a split skin graft but this does necessitate two weeks in hospital for the graft to become stable and the patient remobilised.

Skin avulsion occurs when the arm, hand or hair is caught in unguarded machinery. Occasionally this can be replaced successfully by microsurgery but more usually the skin is damaged beyond replacement and the defect is covered with a split skin graft. If a tendon, bone or joint is exposed a flap will be necessary.

De-gloving injuries occur in the limbs or lower trunk from a run-over accident by a heavy vehicle. The skin is torn off the limb or trunk over a large area and although it may remain in place it is separated from its blood supply and quickly dies of ischaemia. The skin is stretched and crushed and attempts to replace it almost always result in failure.

Surgical procedure

In all the types of skin loss mentioned above, the first essential is to examine the wound thoroughly under a general anaesthetic, removing all devitalised tissue and covering the defect with a split skin graft unless there is exposure to bare cortical bone, tendon or open joint. It is permissible to delay the skin grafting for 48 hours to check that there is no further necrosis of tissue.

Nursing care

The patient with a severe de-gloving injury will be shocked and must be managed as described in Chapter 7.

Scrupulous attention to all pressure areas is essential and the patient encouraged to take a full nutritious diet and adequate fluids. Immediately following surgery the affected limb should be elevated and its colour, temperature and sensation observed and recorded at regular intervals.

Exposed grafts are carefully cleansed and any special positioning of the patient maintained. Occlusive dressings will be changed on the instructions of the surgeon. These patients will need reassurance and support.

In extensive injury recovery is often a slow procedure and the patient easily becomes discouraged. Calm confident reassurance by the nurse will do much to relieve apprehension and doubt.

Physiotherapy

The aim of treatment is to obtain and keep the range of movement and as much muscle power as possible. Active exercises are given to the injured limb as soon as skin grafts have taken, at 10 days. Once the graft has stabilised, swinging of the limb and walking with support pressure bandage will commence. A walking aid may be necessary. When de-gloving injuries are accompanied by a fracture, active and passive exercises are given, depending on the splintage.

Resisted exercises to the uninjured leg and general maintenance exercises should be given throughout the patient's stay.

ANIMAL OR HUMAN BITES

These are chiefly found on the face. The missing tissue is not usually suitable for replacement. Local flaps or full thickness skin grafts give the best cosmetic appearance. Tetanus prophylaxis and antibiotic cover is advisable.

CHAPTER SEVEN

Burns and Scalds

Burns result from dry heat and among the causes are matches, contact with hot surfaces, electric current and house fires.

Scalds are produced by moist heat. The common causes are boiling water, tea and other beverages, hot fat and steam.

FIRST AID

In small burns where there is no danger of shock the affected part is immersed in cold water, placed under a running tap or a cold compress is applied. Cold water treatment should continue until the pain has been relieved, after at least 10 minutes. A dressing can then be applied. This emergency treatment is *not* to be undertaken in the case of extensive burns. In severe burns the affected area is covered with clean smooth material, for example, a sheet or a towel and the patient transferred to hospital as soon as possible. Remove heat-retaining clothing as fast as possible particularly in children with scalds.

BURNS SHOCK

Heat dilates the blood vessels (erythema) and increases their permeability so that fluid and protein are lost from the circulation and there is venous stasis. Much of this fluid passes into the tissues, causing oedema. Some is lost from the surface of the skin as exudate or into the skin as blisters. This loss of fluid from the circulation causes shock. Most of the fluid lost takes place in the first 48 hours after the burn.

The volume of fluid lost is related to the percentage of body surface burned and not to the depth of burn. Wallace's Rule of Nine is used to calculate the area of the burn (Fig. 7/1). In this method the body surface is divided into sections, using the digit 9.

Head and neck – 9%
Front of trunk – 18%
Back of trunk – 18%
Right arm – 9%
Left arm – 9%
Right lower limb – 18%
Left lower limb – 18%
Genitalia – 1%

The palm of the hand is 1% of the surface area of the body.

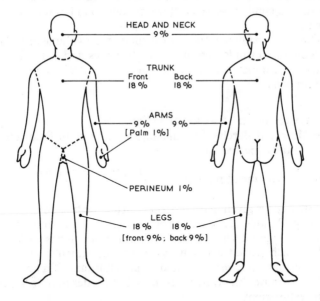

Fig. 7/1   Wallace's Rule of Nine

Treatment

The aim of treatment during the first 48 hours is to maintain the blood volume by replacing fluid at the same time as it is leaking out of the circulation. In relatively minor burns (under 10 per cent in children and 15 per cent in adults) the patient may be able to compensate for this loss by drinking extra fluid. The intake should be accurately measured and charted and a careful watch kept on the patient's urine output. The patient is observed closely and any change in appearance or behaviour, such as restlessness, noted and reported immediately.

In major burn injuries oral fluid replacement alone will not be adequate and intravenous therapy will be needed. The type of fluid administered intravenously varies. Plasma or plasma protein fraction (PPF) or Dextran can be used. Many surgeons consider it advisable to give whole blood at some time during the shock phase in order to combat the red cell destruction found in full thickness burns.

There are many methods of calculating the volume of fluid replacement. Formulae are only rough guides and clinical observations and measurements are essential to control the restoration of fluid balance.

MUIR AND BARCLAY FORMULA (Fig. 7/2)
The Muir and Barclay formula adjusts the rate of fluid replacement to the expected loss.

$$\text{volume of fluid} = \frac{\text{weight in kilos} \times \% \text{ burn}}{2}$$

This volume is given in each period during the first 36 hours after burning. Periods 1, 2 and 3 are of 4 hours; periods 4 and 5 are of 6 hours; and period 6 is 12 hours. A clinical evaluation is made at the end of each period and any necessary adjustments made. The urine output must be 50ml/hour in an adult, and 20ml/hour in a child. An indwelling catheter is inserted in order to have accurate urine estimations.

In addition to the fluid for burns resuscitation the patient is given the normal daily fluid requirements by mouth if possible, or in the form of intravenous dextrose. He is also given antibiotics and tetanus toxoid.

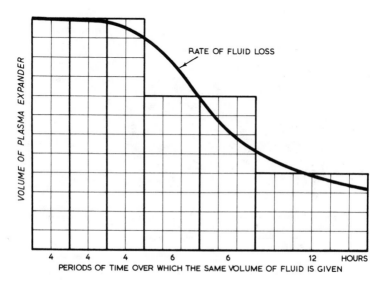

Fig. 7/2 Graph of fluid loss and replacement

Healing of the burnt surface

The depth of skin damage governs the healing (Fig. 7/3).

PARTIAL SKIN LOSS
Where hair follicles, sebaceous and sweat glands remain in the dermis, healing is by spread of epithelium from these structures over the surface.

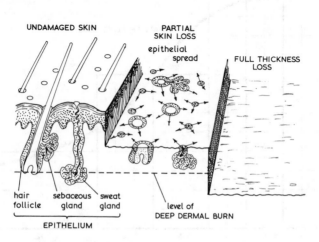

Fig. 7/3   Skin damage following different depths of burn surface.

FULL THICKNESS LOSS
Wound contraction and epithelium spreading from the edge is the only way an area of full thickness loss can heal. These processes are insufficient to heal a large burn area.

DEEP DERMAL BURN
A third category of burn is recognised. A partial thickness burn where the damage extends so far down through the dermis that there are few hair follicles and glands left to provide epithelium,

will heal very slowly and with much scarring. These are called deep dermal burns.

Diagnosis of depth of burn

Partial skin loss or superficial burns occur after the application of relatively low temperatures such as occur with scalds. The appearance is of erythema which blanches on pressure and blistering. The patient will feel pin prick.

Deep dermal burn has a dead white appearance. Such burns are associated with a longer application of a higher temperature heat, typically when a woollen garment is left on a child that has been scalded. These burns are insensitive to pin prick.

Full thickness burns have a leathery or charred appearance, and thrombosed vessels can be seen deep to the skin.

MANAGEMENT OF BURN SURFACE

Partial thickness burns

These will heal on their own provided they are not traumatised further and do not become infected. As it heals the burn is protected by a dressing, or, alternatively, it is exposed in a dry clean environment, when a crust or eschar will form on the surface of the burn and protect it. This crust will lift off when healing is complete underneath.

Full thickness burn

A full thickness burn should be excised and grafted soon after the injury (within 4 days). It is often not possible with very extensive burns, where the burn is mixed, that is partial and full thickness, or the patient is not well enough to withstand surgery. Under these circumstances a dressing or exposure treatment is carried out until three weeks when the burn is desloughed and grafted.

Deep dermal burns

These are best managed by early excision and grafting but the excision is carried out in a special way: taking layer upon layer off until a bleeding surface is reached. This is called *tangential* excision. Skin grafts are applied to this surface. A minor disadvantage of this method is a development of dermal cysts some weeks later.

Split skin grafts taken from the patient's own body (autografts) are ideal. With a large burn, donor sites are few and the amount of available skin limited. The grafts can be made to go further by meshing and expanding. This also allows infection or haematoma to be released without lifting off the graft. If thin split skin grafts are used, the donor sites will be healed and ready for a further crop of grafts to be taken in about three weeks. During this time homograft (skin taken from another person) or cadaver grafts (skin taken from a dead body) can be used. These grafts 'take' but are rejected at about three weeks. Pigskin can also be used and will 'take', but freeze-dried pigskin, which is taken off the shelf, is dead and won't 'take' and has to be changed regularly.

NURSING CARE

Preparation for the patient

Advance warning of the arrival of a burns case is not always possible but when it is, the following preparations should be made:

1. The reception room should be warmed to a temperature of 35°C, and a space blanket should be available.
2. Bottles of plasma, plasma protein fraction, saline, low molecular Dextran, Dextran 70 and dextrose should be available, warmed.
3. A cut-down set, infusion set and intravenous catheters, and, possibly, a central venous pressure monitoring system.
4. Morphia for intravenous injection.
5. Syringes for blood specimens.
6. Guedel's airway, endotracheal tubes and oxygen.
7. Charts and notes for records.
8. A torch and spatula to examine mouth.
9. Urinary catheter.
10. Nasogastric tube.
11. Sterile sheets on which to lie the patient and to cover him.
12. Dressing packs with large pieces of petroleum jelly gauze, dressing gauze or sterile J cloths. Volumes of cotton wool or foam and bandages.
13. Scalpel for escharotomy (slitting down a full thickness burn in

a limb to release a compromised circulation or in the chest to relieve the constricting effect on respiration.

Reception of patient

1. The patient is transferred from the stretcher to the reception room table or bed.
2. The airway is secured.
3. An intravenous cut-down is made and specimens of blood taken. Intravenous fluids are commenced.
4. Intravenous morphia is given (10mg for adults).
5. The patient's burns are assessed by the doctor.
6. Baseline values of pulse, blood pressure and respiration are recorded by the nurse.
7. A urinary catheter is passed and the volume carefully measured.
8. If the burns are over 30 per cent of the body surface, a nasogastric tube is passed.
9. The burn surface is cleansed and the doctor will carry out an escharotomy if necessary. Then the burns are dressed.

Initial dressing procedure

1. The nurse should wear face mask, sterile gown and gloves.
2. The trolley, table or bed should be covered with a sterile draw sheet or sterile dressing towels.
3. The nurse/doctor should explain to the patient what is going to be done.
4. Cleanse the burn surface gently with sterile warm saline, removing any surface debris and deroofing blisters.
5. Apply dressings as directed:
   (a) Silver sulphadiazine (Flamazine) on J cloths or gauze, with cotton wool and a crêpe bandage.
   (b) Petroleum jelly gauze, dry gauze dressing, cotton wool and a bandage.
6. Check circulation in limbs by colour of fingers and toes.

The following are the responsibility of the nurse during the shock phase:

A central pressure line is used in severe burns or old patients. Readings are taken at half-hourly intervals.

Urinary output. The urine volume is measured and recorded hourly. A urinometer is useful for this. The urine is saved and sent to the laboratory at 24-hour intervals – midnight to midnight – for estimation of total electrolytes, osmolarity, presence of blood sugar and so forth.

Pulse rate and blood pressure. These are recorded at half-hourly intervals. The blood pressure fall is a late indication of burn shock as the body is able to compensate at first. It may not be possible to take a blood pressure in someone with burnt arms.

Temperature. This is taken hourly in the initial stages and then 4-hourly from the second day onwards.

Respiration. Serious respiratory problems following inhalation injuries in burns may be delayed in onset. A rise in respiratory rate is the first indication of problems to come, but an anxious patient will also have a high respiratory rate.

Clinical observations. A patient whose extremities are pink and warm has an adequate circulating volume. If, however, they are pale and cold then the circulating volume is dropping. Thirst, restlessness and a change in the patient's mental state are indications that the shock is not being adequately treated.

Accurate recording of observations is essential to the success of the initial treatment. Good charts, clearly written and accurately maintained, are of great assistance to those responsible for prescribing the continuing regime.

Procedure for change of dressing

Patients with a large area of burn treated with silver sulphadiazine and dressings will need to have these dressings changed every 48 hours.

ANALGESIA

It is not possible to do every burn dressing under a general anaesthesia, as it would mean starving the patient prior to the procedure, which would seriously reduce the calorie and protein intake. For children up to 35kg, trimeprazine forte 2mg/kg orally 2 hours pre-dressing and papaveretum 0.6mg/kg intramuscularly, 45 minutes pre-dressing. For children over 35kg, 5mg diazepam intramuscularly and papaveretum 0.6mg/kg intramuscularly 45 minutes pre-dressing (for a child over 50kg 10mg diazepam can be used). For adults diazepam 10mg intramuscularly and papaveretum 20mg intramuscularly, 45 minutes pre-dressing, can be given.

The use of ketamine and diazepam still necessitates starving for 4 hours pre-dressing. Some units find inhalation of Entonox or Ethrane by the patient on demand a useful technique. Patient and gentle technique by the nurse can do much to cause minimum pain during dressing.

METHOD

1. The nurse should give the patient analgesia 45 minutes prior to the dressing and explain to the patient what she is about to do. The patient should be made comfortable.
2. The nurse should then put on a face mask, clean gown and gloves.
3. The trolley should be laid up using full aseptic techniques.
4. The nurse should cut off dirty bandages and place them, together with soiled pads, into the 'dirty' bin.
5. The inner dressings should then be soaked with saline or heavy scrub and removed.
6. Swabs for culture may be taken at weekly intervals or more frequently if patient pyrexial.
7. The nurse in charge should see dressings at this stage and the doctor must see all *first* dressings.
8. Burns should be cleansed, removing all loose pieces of slough and snipping with sterile scissors where practicable.
9. Dressings should be reapplied as directed:
   (a) Flamazine cream directly on to the burn, then covered with J-cloth or dressing gauze, with Gamgee and bandages.
      or
   (b) Petroleum jelly gauze to partial thickness burns and grafted areas; two layers should be applied to prevent it drying out and sticking. Cover with a J-cloth or gauze, cotton wool and bandage.

10. Finally, the nurse should tidy the dressing area. Dirty dressings should be removed and soiled linen and instruments disposed of separately.

Prevention of infection is of utmost importance. Infection is most likely to be transferred to the patient from particles of clothing and the hands of nurses. Particular attention to hand washing and barrier techniques are important.

Procedure for baths and showers

It is of considerable benefit to allow dressings to soak off in a bath or shower and this helps the de-sloughing and cleansing process. It also makes movement easier for the patient. There is, however, a great danger of cross-infection from several patients using the same bath. Plastic liners can be obtained but great care must be taken to cleanse the bath and bathroom using Clearsol, either 1.5% undiluted or 1 sachet of Clearsol in 5 litres of water, for the bath and dressing trolley, and cleaning the floor with sodium hyperchloride solution at the end of each procedure. Most burns units are fitted with a specially designed bath, of which there are several varieties, so that the patient on a stretcher can be slowly lowered into the water or saline at the correct temperature.

Method: The nurse should:

1. Don clean plastic apron and gloves.
2. Half fill bath and check temperature.
3. Manipulate trolley over bath and lower patient into water.
4. User shower hose to assist in removing dressings.
5. Fill bath.
6. De-slough and cleanse surface of burn.
7. Encourage patient to move limbs.
8. Elevate from bath on to trolley. Gently dry and re-dress burns.
9. Return patient to room.
10. Clean bath and room.

Management of the small burn at home and as an outpatient

A large number of burns and scalds, which are partial thickness in depth and involve only a small surface area, can be treated as an outpatient.

1. First aid treatment with cold water.
2. Cleanse the burn and remove any loose epithelium and deroof large blisters, using sterile forceps and scissors, but leave small ones.
3. Cover the area with petroleum jelly gauze followed by a layer of dry dressing gauze and a thick layer of cotton wool and ensure that the dressing extends well away from the burn edge so that if there is any movement the burn does not become exposed. Hold the dressing in place with a crêpe bandage. Check on tetanus prophylaxis and treat if necessary. Administer simple analgesics such as aspirin or paracetamol.
4. Check the patient on the following day. If there is no leakage of exudate through the dressing (strike through), the patient is apyrexial and he has not got increasing pain, leave the dressing in place for 5 further days. Daily dressings are not necessary and can actually be harmful, giving a chance for introduction of infection and mechanical damage to the spreading epithelium. If, however, there is pain, pyrexia or the dressing has slipped exposing the burn then it is best to re-dress the burn.
5. At 6 days post-burn, remove the outer layers, leaving the petroleum jelly gauze in place. As there will be no further exudate, a much lighter protective dressing can be applied. This is left in place for a further 5 days, at which time the whole dressing can be removed, including the petroleum jelly gauze as the partial thickness burn should be healed.
6. Any unhealed areas larger than 2cm in diameter at 14 days are best skin grafted. Areas smaller than 2cm, except on the hands, can be dressed at 48-hour intervals until healed.

RESPIRATORY PROBLEMS

Patients involved in a conflagration within an enclosed space will have respiratory problems, the cause of which are two fold. First, from the inhalation of hot gases or steam and second, from the toxic effects of the inhaled products of combustion. The use of polyurethane foam in furniture, polystyrene tiles, paints and plastics has increased the problem of inhalation injuries over the last few years. A number of toxic chemicals are produced including cyanides and in any conflagration there is likely to be carbon monoxide. These produce lung damage. Lung damage is suspected if there is a history of burn in a confined space. The mouth, palate, pharynx are examined to see if there is any burn or soot. The lung damage may not be apparent for 24 hours and then it appears with dramatic suddenness and is extremely difficult to treat. Arterial oxygen estimations are the best guide at the moment to the presence of lung damage. Bronchoscopy and isotope studies are available in some centres. A chest radiograph tends to show changes after they have developed.

Steroids, antibiotics, humidification of air and oxygen are used in the treatment of the damaged lung. In severe cases endotracheal intubation and ventilation are needed. If ventilation is likely to be necessary for long periods then a tracheostomy is performed.

The airway may be jeopardised by oedema of the head and neck, associated with burns in this area. If tracheostomy or intubation is likely to be needed, they should, if possible, be carried out before the oedema develops, as such procedures are extremely hazardous at a later stage.

DIET AND FLUIDS

In the shock phase patients are given their normal daily fluid requirement, in excess of the fluids that are given for resuscitation. This usually amounts to approximately 2 litres a day and can be given as normal fluids by mouth. In a large burn, where there is poor absorption from the alimentary tract during the shock phase, it may have to be given intravenously in the form of dextrose.

After the shock phase is over, the patient is encouraged to take fluids by mouth and it is important to keep up a positive balance. A fluid balance chart must be maintained meticulously. The patient should be encouraged on to a solid food diet as soon as possible. His needs are a high calorie, high protein diet with added vitamins. The high calories are needed because there is a massive loss of heat from the burnt surface. The proteins are necessary for rebuilding the tissues but also there is a breakdown of protein to provide calories because of the heat loss. Adequate vitamins are needed for the repair of tissue, particularly vitamin C.

Patients are encouraged to take their feeds normally by mouth. Ill patients are often unwilling to do so in adequate quantities and nasogastric feeding using a fine bore tube is often necessary. In extremely ill patients intravenous feeding may be needed but because of the complications associated with this method, it is not used as a routine. High protein and high calorie diets can be made up using mainly milk and eggs and this needs a high volume of fluid. Attempts to concentrate this sometimes result in an osmotic effect producing diarrhoea. Concentrated foods such as Complan again tend to produce diarrhoea. Mixing of these foods must be carried out very carefully to prevent the introduction of infection. Recent work has shown that this is much more common than we were aware and is a probable cause of some of the diarrhoea associated with feeding. The patient will need a great deal of encouragement and persuasion by the nurse to take adequate quantities and the co-operation of a skilled dietitian to make the diet appetising and yet to contain adequate calories, proteins and vitamins. A daily record of the estimated calorie and protein intake should be kept.

PHYSIOTHERAPY IN THE TREATMENT OF BURNS

The aims of physiotherapy are to prevent chest complications, to aid mobility and to prevent contractures. In an extensively burnt patient breathing exercises are commenced early. If there has been a severe inhalation injury with an endotracheal tube or tracheostomy in place, suction should be performed with the greatest possible care, using non-touch techniques. If the patient is ventilated the physiotherapist may be asked to vibrate the chest while the doctor squeezes the ventilator bag and the nurse sucks out the patient. After the patient has been extubated an intermittent positive pressure breathing machine (IPPB), for example, Bird or Bennett, may be used. These machines are of great value for patients with underlying chronic chest conditions present before their burn injury. Children with burns of the face and trunk easily develop acute chest symptoms but respiratory complications may take 24 hours or more to develop. If the patient has chest burns but no obvious respiratory complication, the physiotherapist must take extra care in her treatment. Expansion only should be checked and no vibration or percussion of the chest given, as this may cause further trauma to burnt tissue and superficial burns may become deeper as a result. If the burns are circumferential full thickness burns, the patient's chest will be encased in a tight armour or eschar and the surgeon may perform an escharotomy. This is a longitudinal incision through the layers of the burnt tissue to allow the chest to expand and so prevent lung collapse from the patient's taking shallow breaths, due to the rigidity of the eschar. Positioning of the patient is most important and both the physiotherapist and the nurse must be aware of this. Burns overlying the flexor aspects of the joints may give rise to contracture and steps should be taken to prevent this happening by applying splints, though application may be difficult in the case of severe burns. Plaster of Paris with Kramer wire, Plastazote, Polyform and Orthoplast are all effective methods of support in an attempt to maintain good functional position of the joints, including the cervical spine. It may not be possible to prevent all contractures but it is still important to make every effort to lessen the problem. The use of boards and splints to prevent foot drop are essential and knees should be kept straight. The head and neck should always be supported in mid-position. Hands should be well elevated. All movements can be encouraged from the time a patient is admitted to hospital. However, when grafts are applied, the grafted areas must be kept at rest for at least 5 days, when the first dressing is performed. This does not prevent the physiotherapist from giving movements to ungrafted areas and this should be continued. Full movements can be commenced after 5 to 7 days.

A feature of burn illness is a mental surrender to apathy aggravated by the necessary isolation. Combined with this is a suppression of intellectual and aesthetic interest and a withdrawal from personal relationships. The physiotherapist's daily or twice daily visits give these patients a regular contact with the outside world and can provide mental stimulation.

The specific and general mobilisation mentioned above may exhaust the patient and it must be remembered that they frequently need rest periods. Time must be spent in encouraging and endeavouring to instil confidence into the patient. They need the maximum reassurance and come to look on their physiotherapist as a source of special contact with the rest of the medical and nursing team.

Ambulation

Early ambulation is desirable. The timing varies from unit to unit but in some cases it is possible to have the patient walking before skin grafting. When ambulation is commenced, a supporting bandage of Tubigrip or elasticated red line bandage is applied.

It is advisable to swing the well-supported legs over the side of the bed before commencing weight-bearing. Following surgery, blistering of grafted areas may occur but it is less likely if the grafts are well supported. When the patient is sitting out of bed, the lower limbs should be elevated.

For several weeks after the burns are healed, a support bandage of crêpe, Tubigrip or elastic stockings will be required to prevent blistering or oedema. Footwear may have to be adapted and this can be achieved by using foam rubber or Plastazote. As soon as the patient is able, he should visit the physiotherapy department from the burns ward for his treatment. This will give him contact with people outside the ward although it must be realised that he will at first be apprehensive and self-conscious. The physiotherapist can play a very useful role in helping him overcome these problems.

OCCUPATIONAL THERAPY

The occupational therapist plays an important role in the team caring for the patient suffering from a major burn injury. In the early stages of treatment, the therapist's role is diversionary; talking to the patient, discovering his interests and supplying self-help aids such as book rests and feeding aids. The occupational therapist can assist greatly in counteracting the feeling of dependency the patient experiences which can lead to idleness, depression or aggression. She can help him express himself and build up his independence. Games may be provided to stimulate activity and at the same time provide exercises to mobilise the upper limbs and in particular the hands. Prior to discharge the occupational therapist assesses the patient's needs for daily living requirements. He may need assistance with dressing and feeding and aids to achieve this must be found. He may require help to accept his appearance and to cope with its effects on others. His employment should be looked into and an assessment made as to whether he will be able to return to his old employment immediately or at some later date.

Suggestions can be made as to how he can be assisted in his old job, such as fitting foam pads to handles of machines. An early return to work is not only a psychological stimulant but can produce a much better function in stiff joints than can be obtained with regular physiotherapy sessions in hospital.

The occupational therapist can be of great assistance in the manufacture of splints. Contractures and hypertrophic scars are two common complications of extensive burns. These problems may continue to develop over the first 6 months after a burn. A burn scar tissue is thick and lacks elasticity causing it to shorten rapidly if not controlled by some form of splinting, traction, pressure or exercise. Splints are used to prevent contracture and deformity and maintain a range of movement. The splint may require constant revision. As oedema settles there is a change in range of movement, the patient's weight alters or there is a surgical correction by grafting. The splint needs to be removed for bathing and the nursing staff must fully understand the positioning and function of the splint so that it can be reapplied correctly.

Pressure garments have dramatically improved the ability to prevent severe burn scarring (Figs. 7/4, 7/5). Research into the

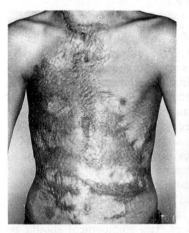 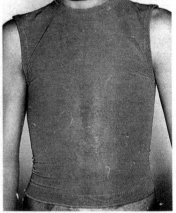

Fig. 7/4   A patient with a healed skin graft to burns of the trunk
Fig. 7/5   The same patient wearing a precisely measured pressure garment

production of scarring has shown that pressure can decrease the rapid flow of blood through the vascular bed, preventing the uncontrolled overdevelopment of fibroblasts and the excessive build up of collagen, characteristic of hypertrophic scarring. Purpose-made garments of Dacron and Spandex material are worn for up to 18 months following the burn, constantly day and night. The scars will then become soft, flat and smooth and the development of gross contractures is prevented. The garments are worn as soon as the scarred skin or grafts are stable. Vests, sleeves, panties, tights, stockings, face masks and gloves can be made of this material. Each garment is made individually for that patient. The occupational therapist takes measurements of the area to be treated, using special measuring tapes and charts. The garment is then manufactured with the aid of a computer. The garment is then fitted to the patient by the occupational therapist, who checks at regular intervals that the garment is fitting satisfactorily and further garments are made as necessary.

PSYCHOLOGY OF BURN INJURY

There is a population at risk from burns. The knowledge of the background to the cause of the burn is helpful in understanding the patient and relatives during treatment. Direct questioning may not obtain the correct answer but slow and careful enquiries by the nursing staff will help to fill in the background.

1. Overcrowded living conditions.
2. The immigrant population in Great Britain are more liable to burns because of the change in climate and need to keep warm and also the change in culture, with unusual cooking arrangements and the use of inflammable clothing.
3. Poverty leads to unsafe cooking apparatus and the use of cheap inflammable clothes and there is often lack of supervision of children because of the need to work long hours day and night.
4. An extra child in the family puts pressure on the economic balance.
5. Illness leads to inability to cope and then to accidents.
6. Marital problems with strife in the family or even diversion produce a climate for accidents.

7. Extra pressure at work allows relaxation of vigilance by the patient or another employee.

As can be seen the patient arriving with a burn may already have psychological problems to which are added other factors:

1. Pain.
2. Isolation. In attempts to prevent cross-infection, we place the patient in solitary confinement, covering our faces with masks.
3. Restraint. The patient is kept in bed and attached to infusions and monitors and the limbs may be splinted.
4. Strange environment. The patient is taken suddenly from the world that he knows to a place with a completely new set of rules and regulations.
5. There is a change in sleep rhythm, with the patient being woken frequently during the night for observation and treatment.
6. Language. In the case of the immigrant population there is an obvious problem, but children have a similar problem with difficulty of communication, which may well not be realised.
7. Some patients may have a feeling of guilt that their action has caused so much trouble.
8. The patient becomes aware of the damage to his body and the likelihood of permanent deformity or disability.

Patients respond in different ways:

1. A few protest and complain. They get labelled by the nursing staff as difficult patients and can easily be punished.
2. The more common reaction is to withdraw into personal isolation and become apathetic and unco-operative.
3. It is not uncommon for adults and children to have a regression of behaviour. Toilet training, speech and manners are affected, and it is difficult for the medical attendants to accept these changes.
4. There is a sense of frustration because of physical disability.
5. There is boredom, which needs diversion or occupational therapy.

The nursing staff will have to deal with the relatives of the burnt patient, who may be horrified by the appearance, and their response may adversely affect the patient. They may be suffering from a feeling of guilt or grief but can react to this in an aggressive way against the staff and they may be fearful of criticism. They too have to enter a strange and rather forbidding environment and are fearful of breaking the rules. The visit to children or relatives in a burns unit may involve a difficult journey and the home and other children are deprived. It can result in fatigue in the near relatives. Mother or near relative can become jealous of the nursing staff because of their inability to help. The slow progress in the recovery of burns can lead to depression in the relatives and anxiety at each operation or dressing is common.

HAND BURNS

Burns at this site are common. The thicker palmar skin usually sustains superficial loss, except in electrical contact burns. Burns on the back of the hand, where there is thin skin, are more likely to be full thickness. The hand quickly becomes oedematous and stiff and the stiffness may remain after the burns are fully healed. The hands are therefore elevated immediately, and remain elevated for some days until the swelling has gone down. Early movements are encouraged. To facilitate these movements, hand burns are usually treated within sterile plastic bags (Fig. 7/6). The moist conditions within the bags prevent the burnt skin from forming a hard scar and the fingers remain supple and the patient can be encouraged to use them. Epithelium spreads rapidly in moist conditions, but there is a danger of infection and some surgeons will cover the hands with silver sulphadiazine before putting them into the plastic bags. A great deal of exudate collects in the bottom of the bag. These need to be changed twice daily in the first few days, although less frequently later. The bags are fitted with a tape or bandage around the wrist to hold them in place. The skin, particularly on the palm becomes white and macerated and looks unpleasant but it will peel off easily; between 10 and 14 days after the burn, partial thickness burns should be healed. If not they will be grafted.

Obvious small areas of full thickness burn in the hand such as occur with electrical injury or a child grasping an electrical fire are best managed by early excision and skin grafting.

Deep dermal burns will be tangentially excised and skin grafted

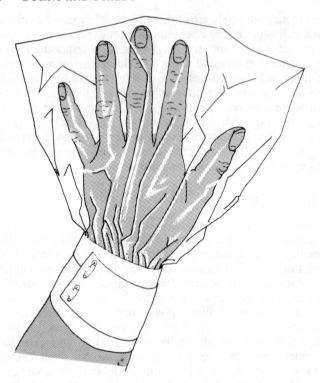

Fig. 7/6 A burned hand enclosed in a plastic bag thus allowing exercises to be performed

within 4 days of the injury. Contractures of skin grafts or healed burns are common. They must be prevented by splinting either with hard splints or with the use of made-to-measure elastic gloves. Sensation may not be entirely normal for some while after the burn and patients must be warned of the dangers of coming into contact with direct heat, for example hot plates and radiators, as well as exposure to the sun for at least 12 months.

Partial thickness burns of the hand can also be treated by closed dressings using a layer of petroleum jelly gauze carefully wrapped around each finger, over the front and back, and hand, followed by a layer of dry dressing gauze, a thick roll of cotton wool and a firm bandage. It is important that the hand be kept in the correct position while this dressing is applied. The wrist should be extended; the metacarpophalangeal joints flexed to 90°; the interphalangeal joints straight at 180°; the thumb should be abducted. This position is the least likely to give a fixed deformity when the burns are healed.

EXPOSURE TREATMENT OF BURNS

This treatment is not carried out as much as it used to be. The patient needs to be isolated in a clean warm environment. Many burns units do have isolation facilities with built-in air-conditioning. The patient is then reverse barrier nursed. For the first 48 hours the burn surface weeps a considerable amount of fluid and needs very frequent changes of bed linen. Frequent turning to keep the patient off the exposed area is necessary. After 48 hours a dry eschar is formed. This begins to separate along the edge at about 10 to 14 days, and on a partial thickness burn will leave healed skin underneath. In areas of full thickness burn, granulation tissue will form, but the eschar may remain attached at these sites for some while. Separation of the eschar can be speeded by surgical debridement or by frequent wet dressings using eusol or eusol and paraffin and regular bathing makes the dislodgement of these eschars easier. Once the eschar has completely separated, and there is bleeding granulation tissue underneath, then these areas can be skin grafted. Exposure treatment is particularly suitable for large areas of the trunk but the movement over the flexures of the limbs cracks the eschar, increasing the chance of infection. Exposure treatment of the hand limits movement of the fingers and is not advisable, but exposure treatment of the face which is difficult to dress produces satisfactory results in partial thickness burns of this area.

CHAPTER EIGHT

Hand Surgery

ANATOMY

The bones of the hands are the carpal bones which form the wrist, the metacarpal bones which form the palm of the hand and the phalanges which are the bones of the fingers. There are eight carpal bones set in two rows: the *proximal* row contains the scaphoid, lunate, triquetral and pisiform; the *distal* row the trapezium, trapezoid, capitate and hamate. There are five metacarpal bones which articulate with the phalanges forming the knuckles at the matacarpophalangeal joints. Each finger consists of three phalanges, proximal, medial and distal. The thumb has two phalanges.

The flexor retinaculum is a firm band of fibrous tissue, which is attached laterally to the scaphoid and medially to the hamate bones forming the carpal tunnel. The median nerve together with the flexor tendons enter the hand through this tunnel at the wrist.

The thenar eminence is the fleshy area of the palm at the base of the thumb and consists of three muscles: the flexor pollicis brevis, the adductor pollicis brevis and the opponens pollicis. The adductor pollicis lies deep in the palm.

The hypothenar eminence is a fleshy mass situated proximal to the little finger and consists also of three muscles: the abductor digiti minimi, the flexor digiti minimi and the opponens digiti minimi.

The deepest muscles of the palm of the hand are the interossei, which fill in the spaces between the metacarpal bones. They insert into the dorsal digital expansion on the fingers and the bases of the proximal phalanges. The lumbrical muscles originate from the long flexor tendons and insert into the sides of the dorsal digital expansions of the extensor tendons. The interossei muscles abduct and adduct the fingers and in conjunction with the lumbricals flex the proximal phalanges.

There are two extensor tendons to the thumb, index and little fingers and one to the middle and ring fingers. Each extensor tendon spreads out as a wide fibrous band on the dorsal surface of the proximal and middle phalanges and is known here as the extensor expansion. The extensor tendon has two insertions, to the base of the middle phalanx and to the base of the distal phalanx.

There is one flexor tendon to the thumb, the flexor pollicis longus, but two to each of the other fingers. The flexor digitorum profundus muscle lies in the forearm. The tendon runs through the carpal tunnel and is inserted into the distal phalanx of the appropriate finger. The flexor digitorum sublimus muscle also lies in the forearm – the tendon runs through the carpal tunnel and the palm at a more superficial level and over the proximal phalanx; it splits to allow the profundus tendon to pass underneath and is inserted on to the sides of the base of the middle phalanx in each finger. The flexor profundus tendon flexes the distal joint; the sublimus tendon flexes the proximal interphalangeal joint.

The median nerve is both sensory and motor. It passes through the carpal tunnel, supplies sensation to the thumb, index finger, middle finger and half the ring finger and also motivates the thenar muscles. The ulnar nerve lies superficial to the flexor retinaculum and supplies most of the small muscles of the hand and sensation to the skin over the little finger and half the ring finger. The radial nerve, which supplies the extensor muscles of the forearm, supplies sensation to the skin of the back of the hand and fingers.

The long flexor tendons are covered by synovial sheaths to allow smooth gliding movement of the tendons. These sheaths interconnect, and it is possible for infection to track up and down these sheaths.

A dense fascia covers the flexor tendons in the palm of the hand. The central area of this is called the palmar aponeurosis and extends from the flexor retinaculum to the base of the fingers where it joins with the fibrous sheath of the fingers and is attached to the sides of the proximal and middle phalanx. The palmaris longus muscle is situated in the forearm and its long tendon runs down to be inserted into the palmar aponeurosis. This is a useful tendon to use as a free graft.

The radial and ulnar arteries join to form the deep and superficial palmar arches and supply the palm of the hand. Digital branches of these arches supply the fingers and the thumb. Each finger has two digital arteries, one on each side of the finger on the volar aspect. The main veins of the hand are on the dorsum.

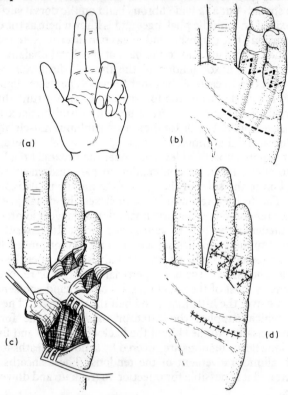

Fig. 8/1 Dupuytren's contracture affecting the ring and little fingers, and the method of surgical removal of the two contracting bands

DUPUYTREN'S CONTRACTURE (Fig. 8/1)

The cause of this condition is unknown but there is a tendency for it to be inherited. It usually occurs in older people and is more common in men. It is characterised by a thickening and contracture of the palmar fascia, causing the fingers to be pulled towards the palm in a flexed position. These fingers can get in the way and, once flexion of the fingers is noted, surgery is recommended. A thickening of the palmar fascia may be present for some years and only slowly progressive. The condition may involve one finger only, or it may involve several.

Surgical procedure

The aim of surgery is to excise the affected fascia, and to restore full flexion and extension to the fingers. To do this an extensive exposure is often necessary, particularly if several fingers are involved. Surgery can be performed either under general anaesthesia or by regional anaesthesia using a brachial block. A tourniquet will be necessary and this can be left in place for an hour while the operation proceeds. The palmar fascia is approached by a transverse incision and closed by direct suture. Single rays and finger deformities are exposed and repaired by a series of Z-plasties. Cross-finger dorsal flaps or skin grafts may be needed if there is much skin involvement. Some surgeons do not suture the palm wound (open palm technique) in order to facilitate early movement of the fingers and prevent them from becoming stiff. The tourniquet is usually released before the skin is closed so that haemostasis can be achieved. When the wound is sutured a firm dressing and bandage is applied. The hand is elevated. The dressing is removed after 7 days and active movements of the hand encouraged. Sutures are removed after a further week. In the open palm technique, the dressing is taken down on the 2nd or 3rd day and re-dressed daily with a light dressing and movements of the fingers and hand encouraged every hour during the day.

SYNDACTYLY

This is a congenital abnormality where two or more digits are joined by a web of skin, hence its colloquial name 'webbed fingers'. It is often found in families, can be bilateral and occasionally occurs in the toes.

Surgical procedure (Fig. 8/2)

If the fingers are joined to the ends, then the growth of one of the fingers may be affected by the other and early surgery is recommended (aged 1 or 2). Where there is no growth disturbance, surgery can be delayed to the age of 6 or even to adulthood. The

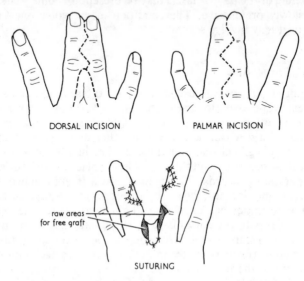

DORSAL INCISION   PALMAR INCISION

raw areas
for free graft

SUTURING

Fig. 8/2   Surgical division of syndactyly

fingers are split in a zig-zag fashion but, as there is a deficiency of skin along the sides of both fingers, it is necessary to insert a full thickness graft. A bulky, boxing glove type of dressing is applied, which provides even pressure and keeps the hand immobile. The hand is elevated and the dressing is left in place for 1 week. The boxing glove dressing consists of a layer of petroleum jelly gauze over the graft, followed by a layer of dry gauze dressing which can be opened out and fluffed to a springy consistency. This is then covered with a thick layer of cotton wool which is kept in place with a crêpe bandage. If the tourniquet has been removed and complete haemostasis achieved, the circulation of the fingers is checked to be satisfactory. The ends of the fingers can then be covered with the dressing. If there is any doubt about the circulation in the fingers, then the tips of the fingers must be left out of the dressing so that they can be examined. It is important when bandaging with crêpe bandages, not to use excessive pressure and pull the bandage too tight, as this can cause pressure necrosis, despite the careful placement of the underlying dressings.

TRAUMA

Lacerations of the skin of the hand are thoroughly cleansed and examined carefully to exclude any tendon or nerve damage and then repaired by edge-to-edge suture. If there is skin loss, without bone or tendon involvement, the defect is repaired with a split skin or full thickness graft. More severe injuries where there is bone or tendon exposed will require a flap repair. On the front of the finger this may be repaired using a cross-finger flap. In this technique the skin and subcutaneous tissue are raised from the back of an adjacent finger, hinged on one edge. They are turned around this hinge so that the raw surface can be placed on the defect on the volar surface of the injured finger. The back of the adjacent finger is then covered with a split skin graft. The fingers remain attached for 2 weeks, when they can be divided under local anaesthetic. More extensive injuries on the back of the fingers and hands or on the palm will need a distant flap from the groin, abdomen or even a free flap.

NERVE INJURIES

Nerve injury may occur alone or associated with damage to a tendon. The nerves most commonly involved are:

1. The median nerve which supplies sensation to the front of the thumb, index, middle, and half the ring fingers and motor to the muscles.
2. The ulnar nerve which supplies sensation to the little and ring fingers and motor to the small muscles in the hands.
3. The radial nerve which supplies sensation to the back of the fingers and hand.
4. The digital branches of the nerve of which there are two to each finger, one on each side of the volar surface.

Good results can be obtained by primary repair although some surgeons consider that secondary repair at 6 weeks is preferable.

The technique is to bring together the damaged ends of the nerve and covering, or perineurium as it is known, and either suture the bundles (fasciculi) or the covering in the correct alignment. The operating microscope is useful for dealing with these injuries, especially in digital nerve repair where the nerve diameter is only 2 or 3mm.

After operation, the hand is dressed and held in a position which will avoid tension in the suture area, either with the application of a plaster of Paris splint or a firm bandage. The dressing remains undisturbed for 3 weeks. Recovery from this type of injury is lengthy. Axons in the proximal segments of the nerve have to grow into the distal segment to reach the end organs; the rate of growth is approximately 1mm a day.

TENDON INJURIES

Extensor tendons

If the extensor tendons are damaged, immediate repair may be carried out by suturing the damaged ends together and immobilising the hand with the fingers in extension for 3–4 weeks. Results are good, active movements being encouraged early.

Flexor tendons

Flexor tendon damage is more complex because there are two tendons for each finger and they lie close together in narrow tunnels in the distal palm and in the fingers. There is a danger of the tendons adhering together or to surrounding tissue in this 'no-man's-land' so that secondary tendon grafting was the technique of choice. Recently, immediate repair of flexor tendons has been carried out successfully as a routine using a precise technique of repair and allowing passive movement with elastic band traction shortly after surgery (see Figs. 8/6, 8/7).

Where a graft is necessary the palmaris longus tendon or plantaris (from the calf) may be used. The graft is inserted to replace the flexor digitorum profundus (the flexor digitorum sublimis tendon is removed) and the graft is sutured into the distal phalanx. The hand is then splinted for 3 weeks, after which active exercises are commenced. Where there is severe scarring of the finger, and it would be unlikely that a tendon graft would run easily, the scarring is excised and a silastic rod inserted to form a tunnel. This rod is withdrawn after some weeks and a tendon graft inserted.

When the splintage has been finally removed, intensive active physiotherapy is needed to regain full function. Despite this, results are sometimes less than satisfactory, due to adhesions, and further surgery or tenolysis to divide these adhesions may be needed.

Fractures of the bones of the hand may be undisplaced, in which case they would need support and physiotherapy to keep a full range of movement. If, however, the bones are displaced, then they will need reduction and fixation. Reduction may be possible by a closed method but operative repositioning is commonly needed. It is difficult to keep the bones in place by external splints, and internal fixation, using K-wires or small plates and screws, is frequently needed. Internal fixation has the advantage of early mobilisation.

RECONSTRUCTION OF THE THUMB

A hand without a thumb is useless for performing any task that requires power or precision, such as holding a pen to write, using fine instruments as in watchmaking or any tool which requires a grip. The thumb may be absent because of an injury, congenital abnormality or removal of a tumour. In an injured thumb every effort is made to preserve length. However, if loss is inevitable or the length is inadequate, then reconstruction must be performed. It is possible to reconstruct the thumb using a bone graft taken from the rib or from the hip, trimming it to the desired length and inserting it into the metacarpal stump. This is then covered with a flap of skin taken from the groin and tubed. It is attached over the bone graft and will need to be divided from the groin at 3 weeks. The post that has been formed is completely without sensation but a neuro-vascular island flap can be raised from the radial side of the ring finger and used to cover the tip and ulnar border of the newly constructed thumb to supply sensation. This new thumb is a rather crude affair and a much more satisfactory reconstruction can be made using the technique of pollicisation (Fig. 8/3). This consists of rotating a finger with its vessels, nerves and tendons and implanting it on the thumb metacarpal. The index finger is the first choice but the ring finger can also be used. The phalanx is joined to the metacarpal with a bone peg and wired into position. The hand is encased in plaster of Paris for 3 weeks when it and the sutures are removed and physiotherapy commenced. The patient will take some time to educate himself to the use of the thumb and persuasion and encouragement are often needed at this stage.

A third alternative to reconstruct a thumb is to transfer a toe. With the aid of an operating microscope the arteries and veins of the transplanted thumb are joined to the vessels in the recipient area. It is also necessary to join the nerves to give sensation and the tendons to provide movement.

REPLANTATION

The function of the hand, fingers and thumb are so important that if these are severed in an accident it is worth replacing them if the facilities are available. An operating microscope is needed, together with a surgical and nursing team skilled in the technique who have the time available to undertake this lengthy surgery. Two situations are considered. First, if the part is completely severed and separated from the body and second, if the part is just devascularised but still remains attached by tendon, skin or bone. If the injury has been a severe crush or avulsion it is unlikely to survive microvascular repair. A functioning nerve supply is essential to the replant and the recovery of sensation in older patients is poor. An upper limit of 50 years of age is recommended. The amputated part is transferred with the patient, to a specialist unit. The severed part is placed in a cooled container with ice packed around it. The reattachment should be performed as rapidly as possible.

Postoperatively the limb is elevated. The blood flow to the replanted part is observed and monitored. The patient is nursed in a warm environment so that the peripheral vessels are dilated. Thrombus at the arterial or venous anastomosis will necessitate re-exploration. The quicker this is done the more chance of success, so vigilance is essential. Difficulties in the blood flow to a replant may occur up to 2 weeks from the time of replant.

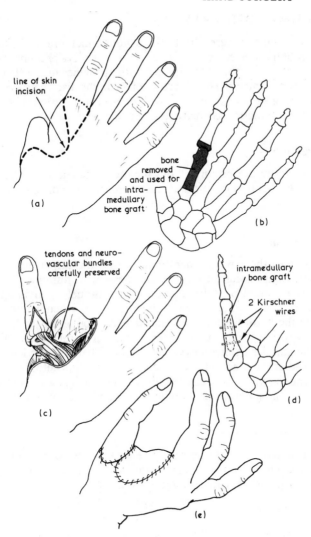

line of skin
incision

(a)

bone
removed
and used for
intra-
medullary
bone graft

(b)

tendons and neuro-
vascular bundles
carefully preserved

(c)

intramedullary
bone graft

2 Kirschner
wires

(d)

(e)

Fig. 8/3 Pollicisation

RHEUMATOID ARTHRITIS

This crippling disease affects the synovial membranes in joints and tendons of both men and women, but there is a preponderance of the latter. Control of the disease is the province of the rheumatologist, but when the hands are involved in the disease process the plastic surgeon is often invited to help. His contribution is prevention, symptomatic, reconstruction and salvage.

Prevention

Synovectomy can be carried out for the joints and tendons. Not only does this relieve pain but it also prevents the progress of the destruction.

Symptomatic

Swelling in the synovial membrane within the carpal tunnel can lead to compression of the median nerve with numbness of the fingers and thumb. Release of the carpal tunnel by dividing the flexor retinaculum can correct this symptom. Rheumatoid nodules in the flexor tendons prevent full excursion of the tendon and may cause triggering of the fingers. This can be relieved by dividing the annular ligament over the tendon. There is a tendency for the head of the ulnar bone to be displaced and this deformity with the synovial thickening can be painful and restrict movement. Removal of the ulnar head can relieve pain and improve function.

Reconstruction

Extensor tendons rupture over the back of the wrist and need repair or tendon transfer. The swan neck and boutonnière deformities of the fingers are corrected (Fig. 8/4).

Salvage

A destroyed joint is painful, unstable and deformed. There are two options to improve this situation: (1) to remove the joint (arthroplasty) or (2) to fix it in a satisfactory position (arthrodesis). If the joint is removed it may be left to form a false joint (excision arthroplasty) or it may be fitted with a prosthesis, usually made from silicone rubber (replacement arthroplasty). In excision arthroplasty the hand is placed in plaster of Paris for 3 weeks and then active physiotherapy is commenced. In replacement arthroplasty immobilisation is maintained for 5 days only, after which special exercising splints are fitted until maximum improvement has been achieved. Patients benefit by regaining function and relief from pain.

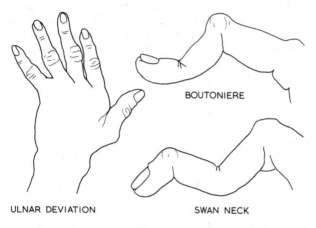

BOUTONIERE

ULNAR DEVIATION   SWAN NECK

Fig. 8/4   Deformities seen in rheumatoid arthritis of the hand

Nursing care for hand injuries

PRE-OPERATIVE PREPARATION

Injuries of the hand are left undisturbed before surgery as interference may cause more damage and increase the risk of infection. Good cleaning of the area with detergent antiseptic solution is performed when the patient is anaesthetised. For the very dirty hand injury Swarfega, a proprietary rapid hand cleanser, is most useful.

In planned hand surgery it is essential that the patient goes to the operating theatre with a scrupulously cleaned hand. Special attention should be paid to the nails, and any hairs on the hand and forearm are shaved. Some surgeons require special skin preparation and if this is so specific instructions will be given.

POSTOPERATIVE CARE

Hand surgery is followed by the standard pattern of care:

1. High elevation with an unflexed elbow. The patient is allowed two pillows only, under the head and shoulders. The hand and forearm are supported in a roller towel or a casing of Tubegauze and these are suspended from a pole or infusion stand at the bedside (Fig. 8/5). Restriction of movement in bed while the arm is elevated is not easily tolerated by the patient and great care will be needed by the nurse to make the patient comfortable. She will need to explain that the hand is elevated to limit the swelling and improve the healing process and function of the hand. The hand is usually less painful if elevated.

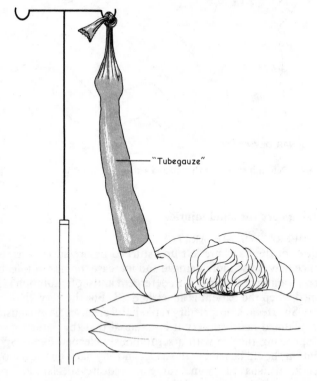

Fig. 8/5   Elevation of the hand after surgery. *Note* the unflexed elbow

2. The fingers are inspected frequently. They are examined for their colour, sensation, swelling or bleeding. Pallor or cyanosis are noted. The 'capillary return' is tested. If the skin is pressed it blanches, and immediately the pressure is removed the colour returns. Delay in return of the colour indicates a circulatory disturbance. If there is any change in the colour then the medical staff should be notified immediately. It may be necessary to split a plaster or release a pressure dressing. Continued bleeding is reported and obvious increasing oedema noted.

   Pain is an important symptom and must be noted. It may be due to too tight a dressing or plaster and might indicate the necessity for release of a plaster or bandage. Pain unrelieved by simple analgesics should be reported to the medical staff.

3. Movements of the hands are of the utmost importance. Once movement is lost it is difficult to regain and in some cases may remain permanent. Light dressings only are applied to raw surfaces so that movements can be encouraged. The nurse should understand the aims and methods of physiotherapy of the hand so that she can encourage the patient when the physiotherapist is unavailable. Encouragement by the nurse to use the hand for 5 minutes every hour will augment the detailed instructions to the patient by the physiotherapist on her daily visit.

4. Patients with rheumatoid arthritis of the hand have other deformities which may make them bedfast; they will need special care associated with their incapacity, and a continuance of any drug regime that was established prior to admission to hospital.

Patients undergoing hand surgery are discharged rapidly and will attend as outpatients for continuing care. The average stay is between 2 and 3 days following surgery. If the operation is to be successful it is essential that at the time of discharge the patient is given careful instructions as to how to continue elevation and to recognise possible signs of complication such as increasing swelling and redness. The patient is given firm appointments for further inspection and dressings and for physiotherapy.

PHYSIOTHERAPY FOR HAND SURGERY

Physiotherapy commences immediately postoperatively, to prevent stiffness of the various joints not involved in surgery. Mobilisation of the affected joints may be commenced at 2 to 5 days though some surgeons prefer to wait longer than this. The hand is placed in a polythene bag or silicone oil during treatment until the wound is healed. Once healing is established massage and ultra-sound may be given to soften the scars.

Syndactyly

Treatment is given in the form of active movements, and in the case of children activities are allowed once the skin grafts have settled. Most children will use the hand without thinking once it is painfree.

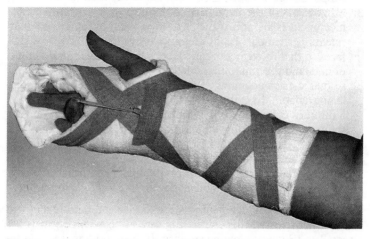

Fig. 8/6 Kleinert-type splint with elastic band – the resting position

Nerve and tendon repairs

Early mobilisation depends on the type of dressings and splintage applied. If the elastic band method is used the patient is instructed to extend the fingers actively and allow the elastic bands to pull them back into flexion (Figs. 8/6, 8/7). This exercising starts im-mediately postoperatively. If plaster of Paris fixation is used gentle active exercises are commenced when the plaster is removed at 3 to 4 weeks. Passive extension at an early stage is dangerous and can rupture the repair. However, at 7 to 8 weeks, passive and resisted exercises may be added to the treatment. If nerves are involved, sensory retraining may be needed. The patient is given objects of various sizes and textured surfaces to feel.

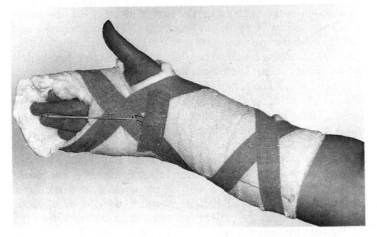

Fig. 8/7   As Figure 8/6 but showing extension of the finger

Pollicisation

Active exercises are commenced when the plaster of Paris fixation is removed. Re-education must be carried out remembering that the new thumb sensation continues to be that of the transposed digit.

Rheumatoid arthritis

After operation for flexor tendon synovectomy active exercises are commenced within 2 or 3 days. Replacement arthroplasty needs early mobilisation and careful direction of movement, using a dynamic splint. Where arthrodesis has been performed the joints must not be moved but other joints which may have become stiff during the period of immobilisation should be mobilised.

OCCUPATIONAL THERAPY FOR HAND SURGERY

The occupational therapist can play a useful role in the treatment of patients undergoing hand surgery. Working with the physiotherapist a planned programme can be arranged providing activities to produce the exercises required for the individual patient.

Disability of the hand makes the patient aware of the fine movement involved in carrying out an activity. This awareness along with the probable pain and fear may distract the patient and deter him from achieving his aim, therefore games and some craft activities are most useful. These help the patient to focus his attention on the end result and forget the disability. Table games played individually or with another patient or member of the staff are very useful. These may include blow football, bagatelle, card games, spillikins, peggotty and solitaire; these all encourage flexion of the metacarpophalangeal joints and the interphalangeal joints, all movements of the thumb, and improve the grip. Games too can increase tolerance and build up muscle power to perfect fine movements. Therapeutic putty, a silicone preparation, is particularly useful for exercising the hand. It is clean to use and by manipulating it in his hand the patient can stimulate joint movement.

The occupational therapist is responsible for making a functional assessment of the hand; a good assessment can assist the surgeon when deciding on future surgery. Assessment is carried out using specially structured forms to record grip, pinch, stereognosis and daily living activities. The flexor and extensor deficit of the hand is measured, the angle of joint flexion and extension, the strength of the grip and the measurement of two-point discrimination and localisation of nerve regeneration charted at regular intervals to show progress and improvement. An assessment test should be structured not only to assess fairly, clearly defined movements, but also to check whether the patient can achieve movement by unconventional means.

Splinting is an integral part of hand surgery and as the occupational therapist is trained to assess hand movements employed in daily activities it is she who will be asked to make and fit a splint. As time is an important factor in the prevention of deformity the therapist and the surgeon have a responsibility to recognise the need for splinting immediately it arises and to check frequently for any alteration to the splint once it is applied.

Splints are either static or dynamic. Static splints have no movable parts. They may be *protective* to prevent weak muscles from being stretched and contractures from developing: *supportive* when they become a substitution for weak muscles and support a joint or arch; *immobile* to keep an arthritic joint at rest or to assist with healing of a traumatic lesion; and *corrective* to force a joint into a correct or near correct alignment and so maintain a good functional position during healing and recovery. A static splint does not provide active stretch but retains stretch that has been achieved by treatment.

A dynamic splint gives mobility to the joint by providing a substitute for absent muscle power. By giving directional control to the joints adhesions are decreased and joint function maintained. Dynamic splints must be carefully designed to provide specific pull with good directional control, using outriggers accurately and securely placed to the body of the splint. It is important that these splints are stable and fit correctly in the position required. Dynamic splints assist weak muscle power and prevent contraction or impending contracture. They maintain balance, promote rest or mobilise specific joints. Good application of dynamic traction provides a gentle persistent force to which scar tissue will yield without excessive reaction over a long period of time. Active movements can be encouraged for the pumping action of contracting muscle will relieve oedema and increase joint range. Where contractures are present 8 hours of light steady tension are more effective than vigorous passive exercise for 20 minutes. Progressive alteration to a static splint (serial splinting) will draw out a contracture and active dynamic splinting will aid in maintaining the correction.

It is essential that the patient and all members of the staff understand the purpose of a hand splint, how it should be worn and for what purpose it is there. However, it is the patient who has the final word in the wearing of a splint and no matter how perfect the design or how effective the application, if the patient rejects it the cause is lost.

CHAPTER NINE

Malignant Disease

The plastic surgeon treats mainly tumours of the skin, tumours of the head and neck, including the oral cavity, and soft tissue tumours of the fascia and muscles. These are tissues situated at sites where repair using skin grafts and flaps is necessary or where appearance is important.

SKIN TUMOURS

There are three types: (1) basal cell carcinoma; (2) squamous cell carcinoma; and (3) malignant melanoma.

Basal cell carcinoma (rodent ulcer) (BCC) (Fig. 9/1)

This is a common locally malignant tumour, which means that it infiltrates and spreads to the surrounding tissues without metastasising (spread to other areas of the body). Growth is usually slow and may take many months or even years to reach an appreciable size. It commonly occurs on the head and neck and mostly in older people, particularly if they have been exposed to sunlight for much of their life. Basal cell carcinomas are very common in white people in Australia and South Africa.

Several types of basal cell carcinoma are now recognised – from the slowly growing 'cystic' nodule or small ulcer, to the 'infiltrating' type which is difficult to eradicate and may eventually kill by eroding into a major vessel or by intracranial extension.

Most tumours are excised surgically with an adequate clearance, or treated by radiotherapy, and the cure rate is about 95 per cent. The smaller tumours are removed under local anaesthetic as an

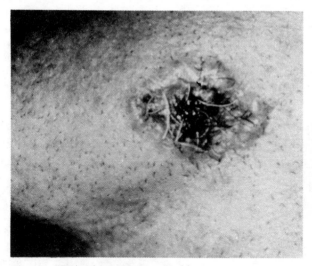

Fig. 9/1   Basal cell carcinoma on the chin

outpatient and the defect is closed by an approximation of the edges, by the use of a full thickness graft or by a local skin flap. Tumours of the eyelid and the alar of the nose may need complex reconstruction. Recurrence does occur and the patient may develop a new basal cell carcinoma at another site, so follow-up for 2 to 5 years is recommended.

Squamous cell carcinoma (epithelioma) (SCC) (Fig. 9/2)

This tumour infiltrates locally but also metastasises via the lymphatics to the regional lymph nodes and at a later stage to the bloodstream and through the body. It occurs spontaneously or as a malignant change in a variety of situations. Strong sunlight for many years produces a change in the skin of old people which is called solar keratosis and this may develop a squamous carcinoma. Squamous carcinoma can also occur in chronic ulcers or in unstable scars, for instance following burns and in irradiated tissue. Some skin disorders, such as discoid lupus erythematosus, old TB and xeroderma pigmentosa are prone to develop squamous carcinomas. The appearance may be of a nodule, an ulcer with a raised edge, or a fungating mass. Treatment is by radiotherapy or by wide surgical excision, depending on the position. If the lymph nodes are clinically involved with tumour then they are removed in continuity. If they are adjacent to the primary, the skin defect is closed with a split skin graft or flap; a flap is particularly useful if the area has previously been irradiated.

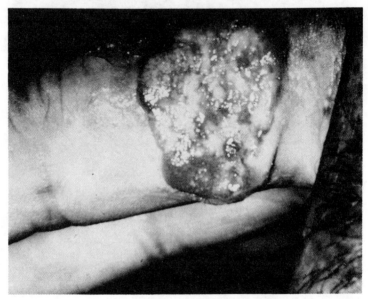

Fig. 9/2   Squamous cell carcinoma of the finger

Malignant melanoma (Fig. 9/3)

There is an increasing incidence of this type of skin tumour which involves both young people and old. Melanoma on the lower limb of a young woman is not uncommon and dealing with young patients with malignancy needs special tact and care, particularly in the case of the breadwinner or child-rearer.

The tumour originates in the pigment cell, the melanocyte, in the basal layer of the epidermis of the skin and may start in a pre-existing mole or present in unblemished skin. The signs to note are a change in size either upwards from the surface of the skin or by spreading outwards; change in pigmentation which becomes irregular or patchy; irritation; ulceration and bleeding. The tumour spreads through the dermal lymphatics to the lymph nodes and then to the bloodstream, to the liver, the bones and the brain and many other sites.

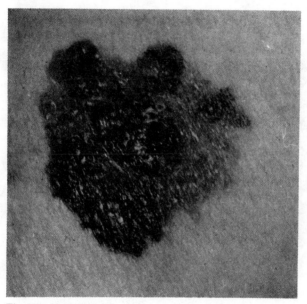

Fig. 9/3   Malignant melanoma

The diagnosis is confirmed by an excision biopsy and treatment is by a wide surgical excision, removing the skin down to and including the deep fascia. The width of the excision necessitates a split skin graft to close the defect. The lymph nodes are removed if clinically involved. The prognosis is good (75 per cent five-year survival) for the superficial spreading type of tumour which is thin and has not penetrated to the deeper layer of the dermis, but nodular growths have a poor prognosis (35 per cent five-year survival). However, metastases and recurrences may occur many years later and continuous follow-up at six-monthly intervals is advisable.

HEAD AND NECK TUMOURS

The majority of these tumours originate in the mucosa and are squamous carcinomas or epitheliomas. They infiltrate locally and may metastasise to the regional lymph nodes. The site of origin can be any mucosa, but the common positions are tongue (Fig. 9/4), floor of mouth, gum (which rapidly infiltrates the bone),

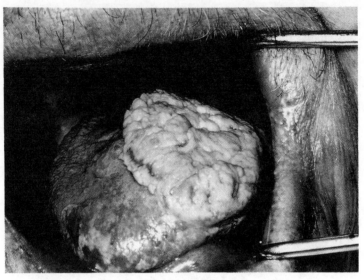

Fig. 9/4   Carcinoma of the tongue

cheek, tonsil, pharynx, palate, antrum and other paranasal sinuses. The tumour presents as an ulcer, a nodule or a fungating growth. Biopsy and examination under anaesthetic confirm the diagnosis and the extent of the disease. Some tumours such as those of the tongue do well with radiotherapy (radioactive needles are placed within the tumour of the tongue); other small lesions can be completely excised and the defect closed either by suturing the edges or by covering with a split skin graft but many of the large lesions, particularly with bone or regional lymph node involvement, require wide excisional surgery and complex reconstruction. For instance, tumours of the floor of the mouth will require a hemi-mandibulectomy and node dissection, a major procedure which used to be called a 'commando' operation. In any one case it may be necessary to provide a flap for lining the inside of the mouth and another for covering the skin surface. The forehead is a convenient and safe flap but leaves an unsightly scar and there are now alternatives to this using, for instance, the deltopectoral flap, the pectoralis major myocutaneous flap or even using a free flap transfer such as a radial forearm flap (See Figs. 4/11; p. 57 and 4/12, p. 58). Repair of the jaw may not be necessary but if it is then bone grafting is used either immediately or some months later. In the latter case a metal or plastic spacer can be used as a temporary measure. Operations on the tongue and jaw may interfere with the airway and necessitate a temporary tracheostomy.

Carcinoma of the maxilla

At this site the tumours originate from the mucosa lining the maxillary antrum or from the palatal mucosa. They are usually squamous carcinoma although adenocarcinomas can occur and some tumours originate from the salivary tissue in the palatal mucosa. Although the palate can be removed through an intra-oral approach the whole of the maxilla can only be approached by reflecting a flap of the cheek and splitting the upper lip. If the tumour has progressed through the orbital floor then it may be necessary to remove the eye as well. The cavity that remains is filled with an obturator which is covered by a split skin graft and is attached to a denture or the other teeth.

Salivary glands

These are the parotid, submandibular, sublingual and many small glands that are present in the mucosa of the cheeks, lips and palate. A *pleomorphic adenoma* (mixed parotid tumour) is a benign slow-growing tumour which can increase to a considerable size. It is situated in the region of the ear. Surgical removal involves dissection of the tumour and removal of the superficial part of the parotid gland, taking care to preserve the branches of the facial nerve (VIIth cranial nerve) (Fig. 9/5). This operation is named a superficial parotidectomy.

Adenocystic carcinoma is a malignant tumour which does

metastasise yet it is slow-growing over several years. An *anaplastic carcinoma* is a fast-growing tumour of the salivary glands which metastasises quite rapidly to the regional lymph nodes and to the bloodstream. Facial weakness results from involvement of the facial nerve with malignant tumour but there may be a temporary weakness following superficial parotidectomy for a benign tumour when there has been much traction on the nerve. The nerve is purposely removed in a malignant tumour in order to obtain a complete excision but it may be repaired using a nerve graft. The submandibular gland is less commonly involved by tumour but its removal may be necessary for a stone in the duct. It is removed through an incision just below the jaw line.

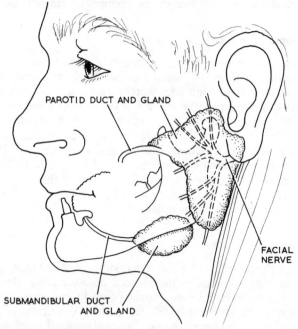

PAROTID DUCT AND GLAND

FACIAL NERVE

SUBMANDIBULAR DUCT AND GLAND

Fig. 9/5   The parotid gland and submandibular gland showing the proximity of the facial nerve

LYMPH NODES

Clearing of the lymph nodes in the groin, axilla or neck is undertaken if they are clinically involved with tumour, either a squamous carcinoma or a melanoma. These operations are often called a block dissection or, in the case of the neck, a radical neck dissection.

Groin dissection

Using a skin incision the fat and the lymph nodes are removed in the femoral triangle below the inguinal ligament, together with the long saphenous vein but retaining the femoral artery and the femoral vein. The wound is closed and the hip is kept flexed for 4 days as this helps in the healing. Most surgeons will use a low pressure suction drain which is left until drainage ceases and there may be considerable drainage of fluid from the leg into the wound. Healing of the skin edge is slow and sutures should be left in place for 10 to 14 days. Deep venous thrombosis is a definite hazard and compression stockings should be worn. It is wise to persuade the patient to wear these for 6 weeks postoperatively, as swelling of the limb occurs. It is not uncommon to have a degree of swelling of the lower limb for life after this operation (see lymphoedema).

Axillary dissection

Lymph nodes are removed as one block of tissue from the axilla, suction drainage is used and a firm dressing applied to prevent collection of fluid or blood. The healing here is not such a problem as in the groin but the swelling of the arm may persist and be a long-term complication. Pressure on the arm using an elastic sleeve and elevation at night are simple remedies; for more complex treatment see Chapter 12 (lymphoedema).

Neck dissection (Fig. 9/6)

Removal of the nodes here requires the excision of the sterno-mastoid muscle and the internal jugular vein as well. Healing of the wound is a problem if radiotherapy has been given previously. Should the wound break down then exposure of the carotid artery is a concern as fatal haemorrhage is a definite risk. Following this operation there is a poor appearance of the neck, one side is thinned and there is a weakness of the corner of the mouth where part of the facial nerve has been sacrificed. The patient also complains of pain in the shoulder as the accessory nerve to the trapezius muscle has to be divided and this muscle is paralysed.

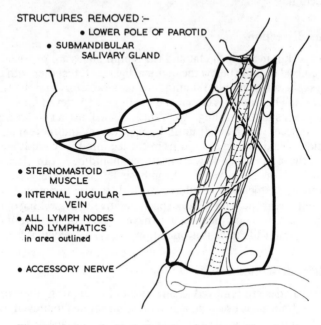

STRUCTURES REMOVED :–
• LOWER POLE OF PAROTID
• SUBMANDIBULAR SALIVARY GLAND
• STERNOMASTOID MUSCLE
• INTERNAL JUGULAR VEIN
• ALL LYMPH NODES AND LYMPHATICS in area outlined
• ACCESSORY NERVE

Fig. 9/6   Incision for block dissection of the cervical lymph nodes

LASER SURGERY

The CO_2 laser is useful in the removal of intra-oral tumours, particularly those of the tongue, as postoperatively there is little pain or swelling. However, the apparatus is not easily available and healing time may be prolonged.

NURSING CARE

The patient attending the ward or the outpatient department for treatment of malignancy may be suffering from a small easily curable tumour or from a fungating cancer which could prove fatal.

The majority of patients will be anxious as they suspect or know they have 'cancer'. There is still a social stigma about cancer and a lack of understanding that many cases can be successfully treated. There may have been a relative or acquaintance who has died from the disease in pain and without dignity. The anxiety may be hidden beneath a confident or jocular manner. The majority of patients appreciate a frank discussion but there are a few who would say 'If I have cancer I don't want to know', and others of an excessively anxious disposition who cannot cope with the knowledge of the problem. Early assessment of the patient from this aspect is desirable and the nurse is usually the person most likely to gain his or her confidence. There is a chance for subtle questioning as the patient's details are taken on admission to the ward and as he is being comfortably settled. Without breaking confidence the information should be relayed to the ward sister and the medical staff. Then there should be a united policy for each patient on what they should be told. Comments from a responsible relative are helpful and the situation is discussed with them.

The initial assessment must take into account the degree of pain, the nutrition, any gross disfigurement and even the smell of a fungating tumour. The nurse must have an idea if a complex surgical procedure needing observation and extensive nursing care postoperatively will be needed. She must also have an understanding of the home conditions, the availability of relations and their commitments so that plans for return home and work can be made.

The patient's treatment is then planned. For instance where should he be placed in the ward? If there is need for intensive nursing after a major resection, he will need to be positioned near the nursing station. It would be very distressing for a patient to be positioned alongside another with a recurrent or inoperable tumour, and a patient with a smelly fungating tumour which could be the source of cross-infection may pose a difficult problem. The plan of medical treatment is sought as early as possible and the patient prepared. Patients with head and neck tumours often become malnourished and it is advisable to spend some while improving their nutrition as they withstand surgery better and the wound heals faster (see p. 185). Reassurance and explanation must be given to the patient regarding the possibilities of tracheostomy, feeding tube, intravenous infusion, suction tubes, dressings and pain relief.

Prior to surgery the operation site is thoroughly cleansed and shaved and this must include any possible skin graft and donor area. It is advisable to check with the plastic surgeon what area should be shaved, as it is important for him to know the hairy areas. A flap from a hair-bearing area placed within the mouth will still grow hairs and this could cause difficulties in the future. Oral hygiene may be a problem pre-operatively if the patient has pain and difficulty in opening the mouth. Frequent mouthwashes with large volumes of fluid are recommended and can be flavoured with Euthymol. If the patient is likely to return from the operating theatre to the intensive care unit (ICU) this should be explained. A visit to the ICU beforehand may be possible and useful. These explanations to the patient need to be done carefully and in a reassuring way so as not to frighten him into refusing necessary treatment.

Care of skin grafts and flaps for malignancy is no different than those procedures carried out for other reasons (see Chapters 3 and 4). However, observation of the flap colour in the mouth is difficult and flaps brought up from the chest appear very pale. Regular observation and recording of these observations is important and any change must be reported to the medical staff. Suture lines are cleansed and supported if necessary by dressings or tape. The surgeon is concerned with:

(a) Haematoma formation which may necessitate a return to theatre for evacuation and haemostasis.

(b) Breakdown of the wound which could expose a major vessel and cause a fatal haemorrhage or a breakdown of the wound in the mouth with the development of an oro-cutaneous fistula. If this occurs packing of the wound may make the hole larger. Resuturing is sometimes possible but the odematous skin does not hold sutures well. Removal of the sutures from the neck if the area has been irradiated and the silk sutures in the mouth is best done using a good light with the patient in a dental chair.

(c) Drainage of the neck wound. The presence of a quantity of milky white fluid (chyle) in the suction drain on the left side of the neck occurs when there is a leak from the thoracic duct.

The patient will need considerable reassurance postoperatively and adequate analgesia. When well enough the results of the surgery are discussed with the patient. An optimistic approach is essential following treatment. The patient and the relatives should be prepared for the discharge date and any arrangements for dressings and analgesia in the home should be made, in good time. These patients are followed-up regularly at intervals for many years in case of local recurrence or metastases. In some cases a combination of treatment will have been required using radiotherapy or surgery and chemotherapy.

Head and neck resections require special nursing care.

Position. The patient is nursed sitting up for some days to reduce the oedema.

Oral hygiene (see Chapter 6, Facial Fractures). Irrigation using a large bladder syringe or plastic squeezy bottle containing quantities of warm fluid (mouthwash or bicarbonate). The fluid is allowed to flow forward out of the lips and into the kidney dish. A soft brush or cotton wool bud is wiped very gently over the suture line. Soft paraffin is applied to the lips to stop them drying out. There is a tendency for saliva to dribble out of the corner of the mouth which is distressing for the patient and causes maceration of the surrounding skin. It may be possible to help this by supporting the lip with tape, otherwise a bowl and a bib will be needed. Apart from oral hygiene the instructions will probably recommend no food or fluids by mouth for some days although sips of water will be allowed after a few hours. Nasogastric feeding will be needed until the suture line is healed at 14 days. A tube is passed either pre-operatively or by the anaesthetist at the start of the operation. A fine bore tube is preferable: it must be checked that it is in the stomach and not in the bronchi by aspirating and testing for acid or by radiographic means. High protein and high calorie feeds (3000 kJ) with added vitamins are given by a continuous infusion with an accurate record of the fluid intake. A dry patient has a dry mouth which is then prone to infection. Saliva is an excellent antibacterial agent and lack of flow leads to infection which may ascend the salivary ducts even causing a parotitis. If it is not possible to get adequate fluid via the gastro-intestinal tract, intravenous therapy will need to be continued for a while. As a rough guide a patient will need at least 2 litres of fluid every day.

Drainage. Drainage of the wound is usually by a tube attached either to a vacuum type suction bottle or to a low-pressure suction pump. A close watch should ensure that there is no blockage of the tube by blood clot and that the clip on the bottle is undone. The tube may be compressed by a patient inadvertently lying on it, or be pulled out from the wound as the patient is moved. The amount of drainage must be accurately measured and recorded.

Respiration. Oxygen therapy, if given, should be monitored and the flow regulated. The tongue support may be interfered with by removal of part of the mandible and cause airway obstruction. If this is likely to be a hazard then a tracheostomy will be performed at the time of the operation; it may become a problem when the patient falls asleep or has been relaxed with analgesics as opiates depress the respiratory centre. When the head falls forward during sleep the airway could become reduced.

Swelling of the tongue and pharynx from surgical oedema or even a large flap within the mouth can obstruct the breathing.

The patient will find it difficult to expectorate because of the altered anatomy of the oral cavity and there is a danger of aspiration of saliva and exudate because of the interference with the swallowing mechanism. Patients are often old and malnourished making bronchopneumonia a very real danger.

Analgesia. Surprisingly, pain following these major resections is not as severe as one would expect, and patients are relieved from the pre-operative pain by the removal of the tumour. Nevertheless, adequate analgesia by injection should be given at regular intervals, care being taken not to depress the respiration or sedate the patient to such an extent that the airway is compromised.

SPEECH THERAPY

As well as being an important member of the cleft palate team the speech therapist is also involved where radical head and neck surgery is carried out. Carcinoma of the tongue affecting either the anterior or posterior section will necessitate some remedial therapy. These structures re-adapt to speech patterns very readily, unless a section of the mandible is removed. Compensatory movements with the lips can produce consonants which cannot be articulated normally following a hemi- or total glossectomy.

Treatment is initiated with lip and cheek exercises which aim for greater mobility and control. The shape and size of the oral and pharyngeal cavities have considerable bearing on the production of sounds. This is linked to the movement of the lips, jaw, velum, epiglottis and larynx. Tension of the articulatory apparatus is of great importance. Sometimes laryngectomy or unclosed laryngeal stoma co-exists with surgery to the tongue. Exercises can then be co-ordinated which do not involve glossal sounds initially but build up sufficient oral pressure to inject air into the oesophagus and thereby vibrate the cricopharyngeal muscle. Where there is much scar tissue present, the elasticity of the sphincter will be impaired and it is unlikely that the voice will be good. When the laryngectomy patient has had no further oral or head and neck surgery, voice can be produced using the above method. As he succeeds in injecting air more frequently the patient is able to produce more syllables; eventually words lengthen, phrases are formed and finally natural fluent speech.

PHYSIOTHERAPY

Patients will require pre- and postoperative physiotherapy. Breathing exercises are taught pre-operatively so that the patient understands what is required postoperatively and also to get to know the physiotherapist. These exercises are continued postoperatively on a regular basis and the nurse can help by encouraging the patient to expectorate.

TRACHEOSTOMY CARE

1. Humidification. This may be provided by a mechanical humidifier, attached to the tracheostomy tube or by the instillation of 2cc of saline at regular intervals and *always* before suction.
2. Many tracheostomy tubes have a cuff which can be inflated. This is useful postoperatively to prevent saliva, exudate and blood trickling down from the pharynx into the trachea. Despite the soft cuff now available, it is advisable to let the cuff down at regular intervals (every 4 hours) so that sloughing of the mucosa does not occur. However, when the cuff is let down there is a danger of secretions from above tracking down the trachea and suction should be available. The cuff is re-inflated after a brief period.

3. Suction. This should be carried out hourly or more often if required. The following regime should be practised:
   (a) Put on a sterile glove.
   (b) Take a new sterile catheter each time
   (c) Pass the suction tube through the tracheostomy tube to the trachea without suction. Release the suction and withdraw the catheter.
   (d) Dispose of the catheter and glove.

   It is helpful if the nurse and the physiotherapist combine so that the physiotherapist can shake the chest to loosen mucus plugs while the nurse sucks the tracheostomy to remove these.

4. Tracheostomy tapes. Flaps of skin from the chest are used to reconstruct some defects in the oral region. The blood supply of these flaps is vital and can be compromised by a tight tape around the neck to keep the tracheostomy tube in place. To avoid this the tube can be sutured to the skin.

5. The tracheostomy wound should be cleansed daily and a new piece of petroleum jelly gauze placed around the tube under the flange.

6. Communication can be a problem and the nurse must not be in a hurry; she should allow the patient time to write down what he wishes. As his condition improves he can be shown how to make himself heard by blocking the end of the tracheostomy tube with the finger or a valve tube can be fitted.

7. Silver tubes can be used if a cuff is unnecessary. These have an inner tube which is withdrawn and thoroughly cleansed every six hours.

8. A tube that is blocked and cannot be cleared by suction *must* be changed. Tubes can also become displaced. A spare sterile tracheostomy set, together with a tracheal dilator should be kept in readiness at the patient's bedside.

INCURABLE MALIGNANT DISEASE

The intra-oral tumour which is incurable can be a great test of nursing skill. The problem is one of pain, a foul-smelling mouth and either dribbling of saliva from the mouth or a leak from an oro-cutaneous fistula. The patient may be unable to swallow and slowly starves to death. This should not be allowed to occur and the patient must be enabled to die with dignity and pain free.

Pain relief

This is of prime importance. Analgesics are given not on demand but at regular and frequent intervals so that the patient does not experience peaks of pain. All analgesics may be difficult to take and injections and rectal administration may be needed. The use of a small pump for analgesic injection has been found useful. Useful oral analgesics include slow release morphine, morphine sulphate elixir or diamorphine. For dressing changes or other painful procedures dextromoramide may be used. If possible the patient should remain wakeful, despite analgesia.

Smell

The mouth should be washed out frequently with Euthymol solution which has a pleasant smell and there should be available a scent spray or Airwick on the patient's locker. Sometimes reduction in the tumour mass can help a great deal. This can be done with conventional surgery or by laser, if it is available.

Swallowing

A fine bore nasogastric tube can be of great assistance in feeding the patient, but there is still often the problem of dribbling saliva and this is difficult to control. Absorbent material such as a Tampax can help if it is used to plug the fistula.

Social intercourse

If possible patients should not be pushed to the far end of the ward but encouraged to meet and talk with other patients. Frequent but short visits by relatives and friends are helpful.

CHAPTER TEN

Cosmetic Surgery

The use of the art of surgery for cosmetic purposes is sometimes criticised, yet the beneficial results of cosmetic surgery and the improved quality of life for the patient amply justify its use. There is difficulty in defining cosmetic surgery: 'imitating or restoring normal appearance' is an accurate description but rather wide, so that it includes not only scar revisions, cleft lip and repair but also face lift. An attempt to narrow the definition by the use of the term aesthetic surgery (surgery to beautify) has complicated the issues; some procedures such as breast reduction are less a problem of cosmesis and more one of comfort as the weight of an overlarge bust can cause backache, and sweat rashes (intertrigo) underneath the breasts are common.

The nurse must look at the problem as it concerns the patient and the reasons why the individual is seeking cosmetic surgery.

A person with an obvious deformity, whether this is an ugly nose, a prominent scar or protruding ears, may suffer from the rude comments and even the friendly teasing of others. An apparent trivial deformity can cause great unhappiness and the patient imagines that others are aware of the stigma and are making derogatory comments. How one sees oneself (body image) does not necessarily equate with how others see one. Disturbance of this body image may be serious enough to turn a person into a recluse. Successful corrective surgery can assist these patients in gaining confidence.

Some personal feature may be blamed for failure at work or in marriage and treatment is sought in the hope that it will improve the future prospects. Surgery for such patients who are sometimes described as 'inadequate personalities' is rarely helpful, they usually find fault with the treatment or latch on to another feature that requires correction.

Patients with mental illness such as anxiety states or psychoses are rarely helped by surgery. Psychotics may be deluded about their personal appearance.

The staff should find out as much as possible about the patient's background and the reasons for seeking cosmetic surgery. A critical attitude must be avoided. A patient with a correctable blemish may fear criticism for seeking surgery for vanity. The patient will often confide in the nurse details of his life and background, which explain his desire for treatment. This information may be crucial to the successful handling of the patient and when appropriate the information should be given in confidence to the surgical team. For instance, the nurse's assessment may show that the patient has an unrealistic expectation of the results of surgery and may need further counselling. The nurse on observing the whole patient problem will soon recognise the patient who will need support in the postoperative period and when he has left hospital.

The nurse should be aware that many patients undergoing cosmetic surgery feel guilt when in a ward full of patients undergoing reconstructive surgery because they are taking up a precious bed and using nursing skills. Postoperatively it is common for these patients, instead of feeling elation that the desired surgery has been completed, to feel depressed but usually this reaction is short lived.

BREAST REDUCTION (Reduction mammoplasty)
(Fig. 10/1)

Grossly enlarged breasts are a source of great embarrassment and their weight may give rise to much discomfort. They can cause aching shoulders and back through a stooping posture. There may be permanent discolouration over the shoulders from rubbing of the brassière straps and inflammation of the inframammary folds (intertrigo) occurs.

The surgery is best carried out in the middle of the menstrual cycle as the operative site bleeds less. The patient is admitted the day before surgery and blood is cross-matched, and photographs are taken. The patient baths before the surgeon marks out the breasts. For this the patient will need to be sitting out of bed with

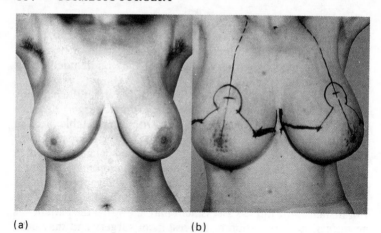

(a)   (b)

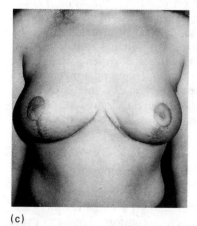

Fig. 10/1 Breast reduction:
(a) before surgery;
(b) pre-operative marking;
(c) final result

(c)

her top uncovered but wearing pants. The surgeon will need a marking pen, tape measure and a pattern. Most patients are embarrassed by this exposure of their deformity and appreciate kind words and support from the nurse. A careful explanation is given to the patient about the likely outcome of surgery and she is warned that permanent scarring will remain.

There are many surgical techniques but most involve removing skin, fat and breast tissue from the lower half of the breast, elevating the nipple to a higher level on a vascular pedicle from which the skin has been shaved. A scar is left around the areola and down to and along the submammary groove, as an inverted 'T'. Drains are used, one on each side and a bulky dressing of gauze and cotton wool which is held in place by a crêpe bandage, Netelast or a many-tailed bandage. The patient is more comfortable nursed in a sitting up position as soon as the blood pressure allows and there will be less swelling. Intramuscular analgesia using 10mg papaveretum will be needed during the first 24 hours, but after this oral analgesia should be sufficient. The patient sits out in a chair on the first postoperative day. The drains can be removed at 48 hours, whereupon the patient becomes more mobile. The dressings are lightened at this stage but the breasts will still need firm support. The nipple sutures are removed at 5 days and the rest of the sutures at 12. It is important to continue firm support with a well-fitting brassière (obtained by the patient) which is worn day and night for at least a month.

Breast feeding after reduction mammoplasty may not be possible. It depends on the type of operation, the amount of breast tissue left and whether it is connected to the nipple. Patients must be warned about this feature prior to surgery. Wound dehiscence and infection occasionally occur. The nipples may be anaesthetic after this operation and vascular necrosis of the nipple occurs rarely.

In extremely large breasts the nipple and areola are best removed and laid on the new site as a free graft.

BREAST AUGMENTATION (Fig. 10/2)

Failure to develop a bust (aplasia) or inadequate breast development (hypoplasia) can be a cause of great concern and feeling of inferiority. In rare cases a normal bust will develop on one side with

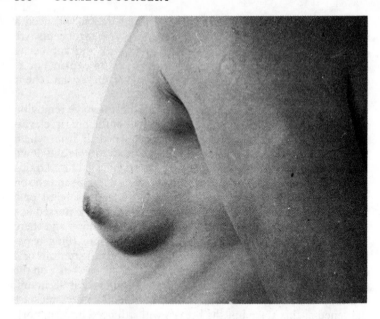

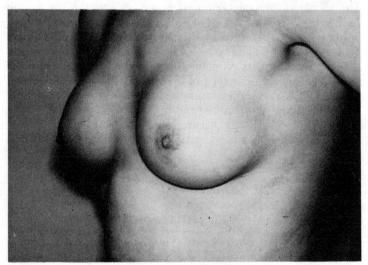

Fig. 10/2 Breast augmentation: (above) before surgery; (below) after surgery

little or no breast development on the other. This condition is often associated with an absence of the pectoralis major muscle and is called Poland's syndrome. Severe breast atrophy may occur after childbirth.

The current surgical technique to augment a breast is to use silicone implants inserted behind the breast tissue or beneath the pectoralis major muscle. The implants are bags, either prefilled with silicone gel to a variety of sizes, or filled with saline at the time of operation through a valve. The implants are introduced through an incision in the inframammary sulcus or less commonly via an areolar or axillary incision. Silicone injections are never used. Many of the implants appear too firm some months after surgery and this is because the body forms a tight capsule of scar tissue around.

Usually the wounds have drains inserted and a firm support dressing is applied. The drains are removed after 24 or 48 hours and the sutures at 1 week. Firm support with a well fitting brass-ière is continued for several weeks and the patient is warned against heavy lifting for 4 weeks after the operation.

BREAST RECONSTRUCTION FOLLOWING MASTECTOMY (Fig. 10/3)

Techniques have improved and attitudes on the advisability of this surgery have changed over the recent years so many more surgical corrections are now performed. Some surgeons reconstruct the breast at the time of mastectomy but most delay reconstruction for 1 or 2 years until the chance of local recurrence is less. Silicone implants are used but frequently there is considerable scarring and thin skin which will break down over the implant. Skin and muscle flaps are therefore constructed to cover the prosthesis and the most commonly used technique is the transfer of a latissimus dorsi myocutaneous flap (see Fig. 4/12, p. 58).

If pre-malignant changes are suspected in both breasts then a subcutaneous mastectomy removes virtually all the breast tissue and the patient can be given a semblance of a breast by introducing silicone implants.

GYNAECOMASTIA

Enlargement of the male breast may occur quite spontaneously in

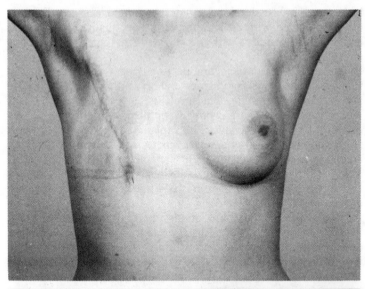

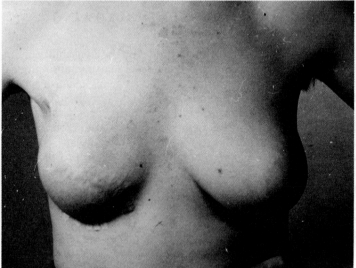

Fig. 10/3   Breast reconstruction following mastectomy: (above) before reconstruction; (below) final result

young men and result in much teasing and embarrassment for the person concerned. Breast enlargement may occur in males as a result of treatment, for instance when carcinoma of the prostate is treated with oestrogens. The breast tissue can usually be removed through a small circumareolar incision.

ABDOMINOPLASTY

Two very different types of patient can be helped by abdomino-plasty. First, there is the small thin lady who has had one or more large babies and is left with stretch marks and wrinkled abdominal skin ('prune-skin' belly) (Fig. 10/4). It is quite a simple matter to

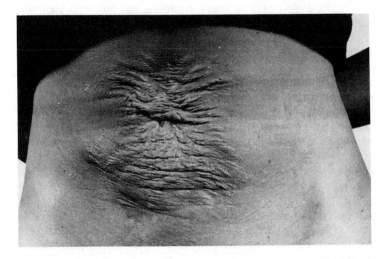

Fig. 10/4 'Prune-skin' belly suitable for abdominoplasty

remove the wrinkled skin, advancing the skin in the upper part of the abdomen, down to a transverse skin at the bikini line. The umbilicus which is left attached to the abdominal wall is brought out at a new site. Second, there is the overweight male or female who has a large apron of skin and fat. Weight reduction which is an important preparation for surgery leaves a massive fold of loose skin. The skin and fat are trimmed off leaving a transverse lower abdominal scar. The umbilicus is preserved, except in the very obese patients. Blood loss may be considerable in these very fat patients and so the patient's blood is cross-matched and the wound is drained postoperatively. A firm dressing is applied and the patient returns to the ward in a partial sitting position with pillows underneath the knees to keep the hips flexed and tension off the suture line. Over the next few days this position is gradually changed, the legs and the knees are straightened and the patient mobilised as soon as possible. Patients who are overweight find difficulty in mobilising quickly particularly if they have a lot of pain and discomfort. The physiotherapist will need to assist in this mobilisation, ensuring that an upright posture is soon obtained. There is a danger of deep vein thrombosis and pulmonary embolism, but haematoma formation, wound infection and poor healing are also commonplace. Such patients put heavy demands on the nursing staff and three nurses are often required to lift them for toilet purposes which they find difficult in performing on their own. Strict attention to all pressure areas is essential. A reducing diet should be continued while patients are in hospital and they are encouraged to adhere to the diet when they have been discharged. Sutures are removed at 10 to 14 days and a firm pressure dressing should be applied thereafter.

LIPECTOMIES

Excess fat and skin can be removed from other parts of the body such as the arms, thighs and buttocks but the scars that remain are frequently disliked by the patients so these procedures are of limited value.

Fat suction or lipohexus is a new technique which is gaining favour and may become a routine part of the plastic surgeon's repertoire. Metal tubes, 1cc diameter and 40cm long, are introduced into the fatty area through a small incision and attached to a high pressure vacuum pump. Globules of fat can be removed from localised areas. Some surgeons first inject hyaluronidase and adrenaline in saline (so called wet technique), others omit this preparation (so called dry technique).

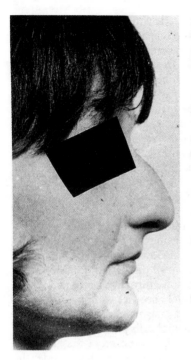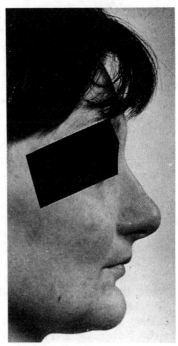

Fig. 10/5   Corrective rhinoplasty: (*left*) before surgery;
(*right*) after surgery

CORRECTIVE RHINOPLASTY (Fig. 10/5)

Nasal deformities either occur as the result of facial trauma or are
endowed. The appearance of the whole or various parts may be too
big, crooked or deficient. Associated deformities of the septum
obstruct the breathing (airway).

Operation is avoided if there is upper respiratory tract infection
but otherwise there is no special pre-operative preparation. All
patients are photographed prior to surgery. The operation is
usually performed under a general anaesthetic but local anaes-

thesia can be used. An incision is made within the nostrils and the skin elevated from the bony and cartilaginous skeleton. The bridge line hump can be lowered by removing it with a bone chisel or saw. The nose is narrowed by breaking the side walls inward and to do this a separate incision is made within the nostrils and the bone divided from the face with an osteotome or saw. Reshaping and trimming of the cartilages at the tip of the nose completes the procedure. The nose is a very vascular area and bleeding during the operation is controlled by an injection of adrenaline, the application of cocaine to constrict the vessels of the mucosa and in some cases hypotensive anaesthesia. At the end of the operation petroleum jelly gauze packs are introduced into the nasal airways and the bridge is splinted using plaster of Paris, a stent or a metal former.

Bleeding from the nostrils or the back of the throat can be a problem. The patient is nursed sitting up as long as the blood pressure is adequate. Swallowed blood can cause the patient to vomit and produce further bleeding so the patient is encouraged to spit out blood from the back of the throat. The patient has to breathe through the mouth and will need reassurance from the nurse. Drips of blood or mucus from the nose are absorbed on to a 'bolster'. This is made from two dental rolls pushed into a piece of narrow Tubigauze and then tied round the back of the head. Alternatively a small piece of rolled-up gauze can be placed under the nose and held on with tape. This stops the continuous dabbing of the end of the nose by the patient which causes further bleeding.

Bruising and swelling spreads from the nose to the eyelids. Ice packs or witch hazel pads applied to the eyelids give relief and lessen the swelling.

The patient can be mobilised on the first postoperative day and the packs are removed on the second day, simply by pulling gently. Any crusts or blood clot around the nostrils are cleared away with hydrogen peroxide and the patient is warned not to blow his nose or sneeze. He is allowed home and returns for the removal of the splint at a week or 12 days depending on the surgeon.

Ether or plaster remover is useful to peel away the plaster and a cleansing cream removes the last vestiges of stickiness. As the patient views his new nose, reassurance is given, explaining that there is still some swelling which may take some weeks to settle completely. Reactions differ: a few people are immediately delighted; most take several days to recognise and get used to their new self even when the shape is perfect.

Once the splint is removed the airways can be cleared by sniffing up some warm salt water. This is made by filling a bowl with ordinary tap water and adding a teaspoonful of cooking salt. The head is bent into the bowl and the fluid sniffed up until it comes down the back of the throat. This procedure sounds unpleasant but actually gives great relief as it clears the obstruction of mucus and crusts.

A saddle deformity of the nasal bridge is built up with cartilage graft, bone graft, or a silicone implant. These are introduced through an incision in the columella or just behind it and bleeding is rarely a problem. However, the bone graft donor site, usually the iliac crest, is painful and there may be considerable oozing of blood. A drain is left in place for 4 to 5 days.

SUBMUCOUS RESECTION OF THE SEPTUM (SMR)

The nasal mucosa is separated from the septal cartilage and then the crooked part of the cartilage and some of the bone are removed by cutting away with a special knife and bone nibblers. Great care has to be taken to leave adequate support for the bridge, the tip of the nose and the columella. Nasal packs are used and removed after 48 hours.

FACE LIFT, RHYTIDECTOMY (Removal of wrinkles) (Fig. 10/6)

Removal of sagging skin and creases of the face helps women to regain their self-esteem. It is a procedure that can also be used in males where the image of an active young executive is the epitome and may be sought by older men facing redundancy. A discrepancy between the chronological age and the appearance can be corrected. Rhytidectomy can also be of benefit in facial palsy and acne scarring.

The patient is admitted the day prior to surgery and blood taken for cross-matching. The patient should be photographed and the hair shampooed. If dentures are worn these must go to the theatre with the patient as they will be needed to be in place during sur-

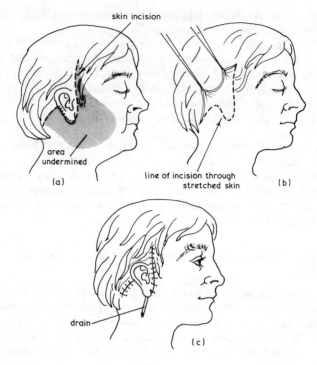

Fig. 10/6   Face lift – operative procedure

gery because they affect the contour of the mouth and cheeks. The operation is performed under a general anaesthetic although in America deep sedation and local anaesthesia are common.

An incision is made within the hairline from the temple to the top of the ear. It then passes down in front of the ear to the lobe and up behind the ear to the hairline where it turns backwards for several centimetres. From this incision the skin of the face and the neck is lifted from the underlying muscles. The dissection is carried down to the corner of the mouth and the midline of the neck. Excess fat is removed and if necessary a tuck taken in the fascia. The skin is pulled upwards and backwards and the excess is trimmed off. The wound is closed. Bleeding and haematoma formation can be a problem and most surgeons use drains and a firm dressing. The operation takes about 3 hours. The surgeon has to be particularly careful to avoid damage to the branches of the facial nerve.

The patients are nursed sitting up to prevent oedema and a careful check is made of the blood loss in the suction drains. The cheeks are examined to see that no haematoma forms. The dressings are reduced and the drains removed at 48 hours. The pre-auricular sutures are taken out at 4 days but the sutures in the scalp which take the tension are left for 12 to 14 days. Patients need only be in hospital for 2 to 3 days but will be bruised and swollen for about 2 to 3 weeks. Make-up is used to cover the bruising after 4 days and the hair can be washed.

The ageing process continues and in 5 to 10 years the skin may have become saggy again. It is possible to repeat the procedure if so desired.

EYELID REDUCTION (Blepharoplasty)

Bags underneath the eyes and excess skin and wrinkles can be removed. This surgery is usually performed under general anaesthesia but local anaesthesia can be used. Make-up and mascara has to be taken off. Postoperatively some surgeons bandage the eyes for 24 hours to reduce the bleeding and swelling. The nurse must be easily available to talk to and reassure the patient. If bandages are not used then gentle bathing of the eyes and application of ice packs help to reduce the swelling and the patient's discomfort. Blood in the eyes is removed by irrigation and chloramphenicol eye drops instilled. The sutures are removed at 4 days but the bruising and swelling may not disappear for 2 weeks.

DERMABRASION (Figs. 10/7, 10/8)

This is a useful technique to smooth acne scarring. The surface of the skin is rubbed away with sandpaper or an abrasion wheel driven by a motor. It leaves a raw weeping surface which heals by the epithelium growing across from the hair follicle, sweat glands and sebaceous glands and leaves a somewhat less uneven surface although the scarring is never completely eradicated. The raw weeping surface is either covered with a dressing or exposed and allowed to form a dry crust or eschar. Healing is complete in

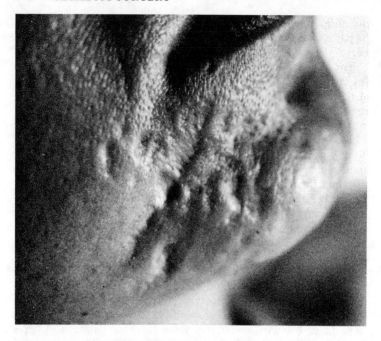

Fig. 10/7   Acne scarring of chin suitable for dermabrasion

approximately 10 days and the eschar lifts off leaving a pink skin underneath. Exposure to strong sunlight is avoided for 6 months otherwise hyperpigmentation will occur. Patients with dark complexions may hyperpigment and a patch test of dermabrasion at an inconspicuous site is usually advised prior to definitive treatment. The dermabraided surface stings and is quite painful. Movements of the face for eating, drinking and smiling are uncomfortable and the face feels tight, added to which the exudate runs down the face and drips off. As the healing progresses the wound becomes itchy. The patient must be restrained from dabbing and touching the raw area and must be encouraged to sleep on his back and not to turn on one or other side, thus avoiding contact with the pillows. The face around the dermabraided area, particularly the eyes and the nostrils, is kept clean with cotton wool soaked in sterile saline.

Chemical peeling is a similar procedure but the surface of the skin is removed by a controlled burn with the chemical, phenol.

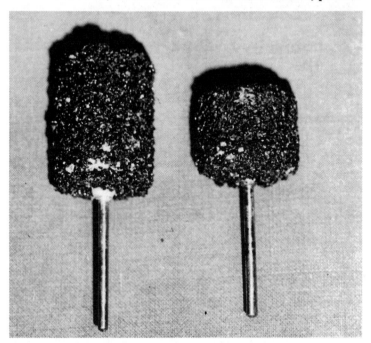

Fig. 10/8   Diamond burrs for dermabrasion of acne scars

TATTOOS

A tattoo is produced by depositing particles of pigment within the dermis. If the pigment is near the surface of the skin it can be removed by dermabrasion or laser leaving a little scarring. If the pigment is deep in the dermis then these techniques will leave excessive scarring. It is then better to excise the full thickness of the skin surgically. For a small tattoo the edges of the skin can be brought together and sutured leaving a linear scar. With a large tattoo the defect must be closed with a skin graft leaving a permanent patch.

CHAPTER ELEVEN

Oral Surgery

The oral surgeon treats a range of conditions relating to the mouth:

1. Teeth extractions.
   These are usually the more difficult extractions such as impacted wisdom teeth (eights) or extractions in difficult patients, for example a patient with a medical problem. Also included in this category are patients with complications following tooth extractions, such as oro-antral fistulae, who are admitted to hospital for correction. Teeth can also be transplanted and replanted.
2. Infections.
   The more serious infections will need treatment in hospital and may involve drainage of an abscess. There is a particularly serious streptococcal infection called Ludwig's angina which spreads from an infected tooth in the mandible to the floor of the mouth and the neck. The swelling of the neck is sufficient to obstruct the airway at the larynx, with possible fatal consequences.
3. Pre-prosthetic surgery, sulcus deepening and epithelial inlay.
4. Cysts of the jaws.
5. Tumours of the jaws and oral mucosa, both benign and malignant.
6. Correction of jaw deformities by mandibular and maxillary osteotomies and mentoplasty.
7. Fractures (see Chapter 6).
8. Temporomandibular joint disorders.
9. Salivary gland disorders.

PATIENT PREPARATION

Much of the oral surgeon's work is on young adult patients, who are admitted to hospital fit and well and are keen to return quickly to normal activity, after as short a stay in hospital as possible. There may be anxiety over absence from work or from important duties running the home. There is need for an efficient admission procedure so that time is not wasted, yet a human touch must always be in evidence. The clinician should have arranged investigations such as radiographic examination and haemoglobin estimation as an outpatient to avoid delay; these investigations, together with dental records and other radiographs must be available.

Some patients who are admitted for minor oral surgery may have complex medical problems, such as diabetes, heart disease and bleeding disorders. Their needs must be carefully assessed and details of any medication obtained. Patients for mandibular or maxillary osteotomy also need careful preparation. They will have their jaws fixed together postoperatively for several weeks and time must be taken to explain to them exactly what to expect and how they will manage after surgery. Patients with facial fractures may be transferred from the accident department or another hospital and not be prepared for hospital admission; thus they have a sudden interruption of their normal life and may need help and advice on sorting out problems.

Operating theatre routine

Operating lists consist of many short cases and can be a cause of errors. The following rules help to avoid this:

1. Printed lists should not be changed in order.
2. The pre-medication times are best written down and not timed from theatre.
3. Ample staff to take the patient to theatre and return with him avoids wasting valuable theatre time.

The large number of cases treated, and their short length of stay, make a five-day ward particularly useful.

Pre-operative preparation

The patient's mouth must be cleaned before going to theatre and the lips covered with lanolin to prevent cracking.

TOOTH EXTRACTIONS

Teeth are numbered as follows:

$$\frac{87654321 \mid 12345678}{87654321 \mid 12345678}$$

The common problem is the removal of the wisdom teeth or '8s'. Human jaws have become too small for the number of teeth they support and the back teeth may fail to erupt or become impacted. Complications then arise. The upper and lower 8s are removed to prevent or treat these complications. Removal can be difficult. The gum is incised with a scapel, the bony side-wall of the jaw may need to be removed or lifted aside to gain access to the tooth and its roots which may have to be divided. After removal, the bone is replaced and the gum and socket closed with sutures. These sutures may be non-absorbable and need removal on the 7th day.

Teeth in the upper jaw may have their roots in the maxillary sinus or antrum. Removal can be complicated by an oro-antral fistula, that is a hole between the mouth and the maxillary sinus. This is closed by advancing or rotating local flaps of mucosa to close the defect. The sinus must be drained through a tube in the nose and passed through a hole into the sinus. By means of this tube the antrum will need irrigating daily by the ward staff and removing after 4 days. The patient must be warned against blowing his nose and sneezing for 2 weeks at least.

Postoperative care

Patients who undergo tooth extraction require only a brief period of skilled care. The patient is returned conscious from the theatre recovery ward and is nursed in the lateral position with the head to one side allowing any blood to trickle out of the corner of the mouth and not down the throat. This is most important as there is danger of inhalation of blood or of it being swallowed when it could cause vomiting. Gauze packs in the corner of the mouth are left undisturbed until haemostasis is established. Once bleeding has been controlled then the patient must be sat up as this reduces swelling.

Oral hygiene in the form of warm saline mouth baths commences six-hours' postoperatively and is continued at four-hourly intervals. There is pain and discomfort in the first 24 hours and effective analgesia should be given regularly. Most suitable for this are 'dissolving tablets' containing a mixture of soluble aspirin and codeine. It is far better to anticipate the pain and give analgesics before the patient feels it rather than have to alleviate it once it has developed. Patients differ markedly in their pain tolerance and it is an important part of the nurses' duty to assess this. It can be done by enquiring from the patient whether he has experienced pain as a result of previous operations, accidents or illnesses and by judging the effectiveness of the analgesics administered.

Swelling of the face after tooth extraction can be considerable and the patient and relatives should be warned about this and told that it is not abnormal. Rapid resolution can be expected – this will be speeded by nursing the patient in an upright position.

Many oral surgeons give prophylactic antibiotics, and lanolin is liberally applied to the lips to prevent cracking. For a simple extraction the patient will be discharged on the day following surgery provided there are no complications such as gross swelling, continued bleeding or pyrexia. He should be instructed on simple oral hygiene and recommended to take a soft diet at home.

MANDIBULAR AND MAXILLARY OSTEOTOMIES

Deformity of both jaws results from congenital abnormalities, for instance cleft lip and palate and also from trauma. In a *normal occlusion* (class I) the upper teeth lie just outside the lower ones, and there is a fixed relationship between the upper and lower first molar teeth. If the lower jaw is set back too far, this is called *retrognathism* (class II). The lower jaw may be too prominent, which is called *prognathism* (class III). Hypoplasia, which is usually applied to the maxilla, is when the structure is too small and there has been insufficient growth. These deformities can cause functional problems because the teeth do not meet (malocclusion) and not only is normal biting not possible but also the appearance may be a problem. The deformities are corrected by cutting one or both jaws and moving them forwards or backwards as necessary. They are fixed in the correct position and held with wires and splints, sometimes solid fixation to the skull via external bars and halo frames are needed. If there is a gap in bone then this must be filled with a bone graft usually taken from rib or hip.

Complicated pre-operative assessment is necessary which can be done as an outpatient in the oral surgery department. Photographs and special radiographs with measurements are needed; models of the teeth are made in plaster of Paris which can be cut and altered, so that there is a precise plan of treatment. In some cases silver splints are cast on the plaster of Paris models and these splints are glued to the teeth with cement in readiness for surgery.

Mandibular osteotomy (Fig. 11/1)

There are several different designs for altering the mandible but a fashionable procedure is to do an Obwesger or sagittal osteotomy. In this, the vertical ramus of the mandible on both sides is split through an incision within the mouth. This allows the body of the mandible to move forwards or backwards and leaves a large area of bone available for reunion without the need of bone grafts. It takes about 6 weeks for the 'fracture' to heal and the jaws are locked together in the correct position while this happens. In other types of osteotomy the approach to the jaw is from outside but care needs to be taken to make a small scar. A bone graft taken from the hip or rib may be used to consolidate the fracture.

Risks. These are bleeding and swelling compromising the airway. The external approach to the mandible is less hazardous but a small scar results.

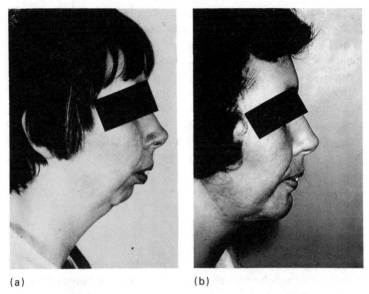

(a)   (b)

Fig. 11/1   Mandibular osteotomy and genioplasty. (a) before; (b) after

Maxillary osteotomy

The maxilla can be cut at several different sites depending on the extent of the deformity. A cut can be made low across the maxilla at the Le Fort I fracture level (see p. 12). The Le Fort II fracture level is used for more extensive procedures. Maxillary osteotomies take longer and are technically much more difficult than mandibular osteotomies and are somewhat more hazardous. Both mandibular and maxillary osteotomies can be performed at the same operation if necessary. The high level osteotomy is approached through a scalping flap. An incision is made virtually from ear to ear and the forehead turned back giving excellent access to the bone. This does necessitate shaving the scalp but the hair will be growing well again by the time the external fixation is removed at 6 to 8 weeks postoperatively.

The bone can be divided at an even higher level but this necessitates opening the skull and a neurosurgeon is then part of the team. These craniofacial operations are performed for rare congenital abnormalities of the face and skull and occasionally for deformities following injury. The patient will be nursed in the intensive care unit for 36 hours postoperatively.

Deformities of the jaw can sometimes be disguised by building up the chin. Although this can be done by grafting on bone or putting in a prosthesis, the most successful surgery involves cutting the point of the chin and moving it forwards or backwards. This is called a *genioplasty*.

Postoperative care

The postoperative care following a mandibular and/or maxillary osteotomy is much more exacting. The upper and lower jaws are fixed together with wires or elastic. Fixation must be capable of quick removal by the ward staff in case of airway obstruction from swelling or because of the inhalation of vomit or blood. Wire cutters *must* be within easy reach of the patient and staff must know exactly *where* to cut. The wires joining the upper and lower jaws are the only ones that need dividing to be able to open the mouth. An efficient suction machine must always be easily available.

Oral hygiene (see p. 97) is carried out regularly every 4 hours during the daytime. This involves brushing the wires, the teeth and all the appliances with a small toothbrush. Regular mouthwashes using weak hypochlorite bicarbonate, saline or hydrogen peroxide are used. If there is any uncertainty about the strength of a mouthwash it is quite easy to taste it before administering it to a patient. A 50ml syringe with a tube attached allows the fluid to be squirted into the back of the mouth at each side so that the fluid with the debris is washed forward and allowed to dribble out into a bowl.

Nutritional needs

Depending on age and clinical condition, patients may be malnourished on admission. Following surgery there may be a rise in the requirements for energy and nutrients, e.g. protein, vitamin C and zinc involved in wound healing. Nutritional status may be further compromised by decreased food intake because of pain, physical interference with food ingestion and malabsorption. Psychological factors and impaired taste may affect food acceptability, palatability and appetite. All these factors may be present in patients having jaw surgery.

Energy and protein requirements can be established from measurements of resting energy expenditure (REE) and nitrogen (N) balance, but neither of these measurements can usually be made as a routine, and clinically useful approximations must be made. Since the prime requirement of the body is for energy, assessment of this is increasingly being used as the starting point in calculating nutritional requirements. REE can be calculated from the measurements of height and weight using the Harris-Benedict formula. This differs for the two sexes.

REE per day
$$\text{males:} \quad 66.4230 + 13.7516W + 5.0033H - 6.7750A$$
$$\text{females:} \quad 655.0955 + 9.6534W + 1.8496H - 4.6756A$$

$$A = \text{age (years)}$$
$$H = \text{height (cm)}$$
$$W = \text{weight (kg)}$$

The appropriate N requirement can then be calculated from the generally applicable ratio of 200kcal per 1g N. Septic patients require relatively less energy with the ratio 180 or 150kcal per g N. Alternatively, the N requirement can be derived from measurements of 24-hour nitrogen excretion with an additional 10 per cent being added for normal non-renal losses.

It is not possible to assess patients' requirements for vitamins and minerals. The recommended dietary allowances (DHSS, 1979) are for normal individuals. Moreover, there are no British values for some vitamins or for trace elements, of which zinc may be of particular importance for surgical patients. Requirements for minor nutrients by patients having jaw surgery are probably at least those for normal individuals. Optimum conditions for bone and wound healing will only exist if all nutrients are provided in adequate amounts. This has important implications when considering the way in which food is provided.

Patients having jaw surgery will have varying degrees of difficulty in consuming normal food. If normal food is consumed it is essential that a record is kept of the amounts consumed so that its adequacy can be assessed. Supplemented sip feeds can be provided as nutritionally complete commercially available complete feeds. If patients can sip these through a straw they should be encouraged to consume target volumes. Since jaws may remain wired for 6–8 weeks, patients may be on sip feeding or indeed on total liquid feeding for much of this time. It is essential therefore that flavours are varied. Many patients can be managed at home in this way. If patients are unable to suck, or unwilling to take adequate quantities of food in this way, they should be fed by a nasogastric tube delivering the feed by gravity or assisted by a pump through a fine bore tube. Bolus feeding through a Ryle's tube should not be used unless the patient prefers a liquidised diet.

As the wires are relaxed and ultimately removed, the diet should be changed from nourishing liquids to a liquidised, soft or semi-solid diet with protein and energy supplements if necessary until a normal diet can be taken.

CYSTS

Both upper and lower jaws are prone to cyst formation. They arise from infected teeth (radicular cysts) or from unerupted teeth (follicular cysts). Keratocysts are another variety that are developmental in origin and have a tendency to recur following removal. A tumour of the jaw called an ameloblastoma may occur as a collection of cysts which are neoplastic in origin. Cysts are removed by incising the mucosa and removing some of the bone of the jaw to gain access to the cyst lining which must be removed completely. The defect in the bone can be left open (marsupialised) or closed primarily. Sometimes the jaw will need reconstructing with a bone graft. For large and extensive cysts, an external approach may be necessary.

TEMPOROMANDIBULAR JOINT

As with other joints this may be involved with osteoarthritis, rheumatoid arthritis or damaged by trauma. The first two conditions need treatment for pain whereas trauma can result in ankylosis, that is a solid fixation of the joint so that the teeth cannot open; the joint is then divided but preventing it from reuniting is often difficult. The anaesthesia for this surgery is difficult because a blind nasal intubation is needed as the jaw cannot be opened to pass a laryngoscope to see that the endotracheal tube enters the trachea.

Recurrent dislocations of the jaw can be corrected by surgery. The temporomandibular joint is approached for the above operations through an incision in the temple and the pre-auricular region.

TUMOURS

Both benign and malignant tumours occur in the oral mucosa and in the bone. Leukoplakia appears as white patches in the mucosa, which grows slowly. They may become malignant after some while. These patches are easily confused with *Candida albicans* infections (thrush) and lichen planus. Careful observation of these patches is necessary as an outpatient and if changes are noted then biopsy is taken and the patches are removed by excision and grafting or cryosurgery. Grafts in the mouth are difficult to keep in place and they are either stretched over a stent mould which is fixed to the teeth or kept in place by multiple stitches through the graft to the underlying tissues rather like a quilt.

Malignant tumours occur at sites of chronic irritation and are associated, like leukoplakia, with smoking and poor oral hygiene.

The nature of any growth or ulcer in the mouth is defined by biopsy. This can often be done under a local anaesthetic but it can be quite helpful to do it under a general anaesthetic so that an accurate assessment of the extent of the tumour can be made, without inflicting a lot of pain and discomfort. Treatment may be by radiotherapy or surgery. Carcinoma of the tongue is particularly well treated by implanting radioactive needles or gold grains within the tumour. Radiotherapy makes the mucosa sore and removes taste for some weeks. It also reduces the secretion of saliva, maybe permanently. This has a deleterious effect on the mucosa of the teeth.

Oral surgery for the most part consists of treatment of a large number of cases of a repetitive and routine nature which necessitates an efficient system. The success of this efficiency can be evaluated by the statistical returns. The human side of the equation must not be overlooked, however, and there must be provision for the few cases that demand very skilled nursing.

REFERENCE

DHSS (1979). *Recommended Daily Amounts of Food, Energy and Nutrients for Groups of People in the United Kingdom.* Report on Health and Social Subjects No. 15. HMSO, London.

CHAPTER TWELVE

Miscellaneous conditions

LYMPHOEDEMA

This condition is due to malfunction of the lymphatics. Protein-rich fluid is retained in the tissue spaces producing a gradual and progressive swelling of the limb. The limb can become so big that ambulation becomes difficult in the case of a leg, and the function of a hand and arm is reduced in upper limb lymphoedema. The skin becomes warty and thickened, hence the name given to this condition, elephantiasis, and there is also a danger of recurrent infections or cellulitis. The abnormality of the lymphatics is either a congenital deficiency or obstruction from tumours and their treatment, trauma or the filarial parasite.

Non-operative treatment is advisable in the early stages. The patient is fitted with a firm support stocking and, if the lower limb is involved with lymphoedema, is advised to raise the foot of the bed at night. In more severe cases it is possible to use intermittent compression of the limb with a special sock and mechanical pump. This treatment should be carried out each evening for 2 hours. Great care is taken to keep the skin clean and supple so that cracks which may start infection are avoided. Diuretics do *not* help.

Surgery to by-pass an obstruction by joining lymphatics to other lymphatics or lymphatics to veins has not proved to date to be of lasting value. There are two types of operation which can be of help. The older of these is the *Charles* or *Macey operation* where the thickened and oedematous skin and subcutaneous tissues are excised all the way round the leg or arm, down to the muscles. The raw surface is then covered with a split skin graft taken when possible from the tissues which have already been removed. This gives a thin leg but wear and tear over several years takes its toll and recurrent ulceration is a common sequel.

Thompson's buried dermis flap operation (Fig. 12/1) is used to reduce the bulk of subcutaneous tissue and to place a shaved skin flap deep to the muscle. This encourages the flow of lymph from the skin into the muscle area where it can escape more easily. The operation is performed in two stages and at each stage an incision is made the length of the limb. One skin flap is shaved (to prevent cyst formation) and sutured to the muscle. The second skin flap is overlapped rather like a Swiss roll.

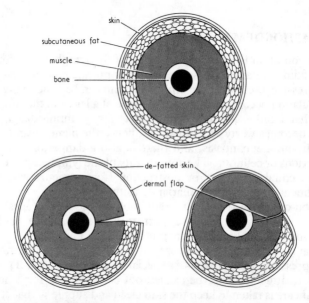

Fig. 12/1   Buried dermis flap

A patient with a lymphoedematous leg needs preparation for seven days pre-operatively. Elevation of the leg in bed for this time reduces the oedema and the tissues become soft and more supple which facilitate the surgery. The skin is cleansed carefully, massaged by the physiotherapist and oiled to make it more supple. The areas of pressure in the involved limb and in the other parts of the body are carefully monitored and the patient moved regularly.

Following surgery the patient will return to the ward with a bulky dressing and the leg must be elevated on pillows and the foot of the bed raised. Two large suction drains will be present in the Thompson's operation, but if a skin graft has been applied in a Macey operation there will be no drains. The drains are left in place for 5 days and then removed; the whole dressing is changed and reduced. A skin graft is left undisturbed for 7 days. Healing is slow but hopefully is complete by 3 weeks when ambulation is commenced. The physiotherapist will teach and help the patient mobilise. The patient is able to leave hospital at four weeks after the surgery.

PRESSURE ULCERS

These occur in patients who: (a) cannot feel or are unconscious; (b) cannot move because of pain from arthritis or surgical immobilisation; or (c) have poor circulation and nutrition such as hypotensive patients or the elderly. Patients at particular risk include the paraplegic, patients in intensive care units and elderly patients with fractured hips.

The ulcers develop over bony prominences, and take their names from the affected sites:

Sacral – from lying on the back.
Trochanteric – from lying on one side.
Ischial – from sitting.
Calcaneal – from not being able to move the feet.

The damage beneath the skin is usually extensive and is present before the skin changes appear.

Prevention is better than cure. Regular turning is of the utmost importance. Wet bedding and rough materials cause skin breakdown: this can be avoided by catheterising the incontinent patient and using sheepskins to lie on. Various mechanical aids such as low air loss or fluidised bead beds are undoubtedly helpful but may not always be available.

Once an ulcer has developed removal of all the necrotic tissue as quickly as possible is essential and surgical debridement speeds the healing. Regular cleansing and re-dressing should be carried out at least twice a day. All pressure at the site of one of these ulcers must be avoided. The type of material used for the dressing is unimportant compared to the avoidance of pressure and regular cleansing. Possible regimes include the following:

Half-strength eusol and paraffin.
Malatex for de-sloughing.
Debrisan.
Jeliperm.
Silastic foam.
Silver sulphadiazine.
Oxygen.
Ultraviolet light.

Once the wound is completely de-sloughed, then the healing can be speeded and the ultimate strength of the wound improved by closing with a flap, such as rotation, transposition or myocutaneous flaps, using the gluteal or tensor fascia lata muscles. The flaps can be used to close the skin defect but it is also necessary to smooth the bony prominence to reduce the chance of further ulceration.

Postoperatively the patient is nursed with no pressure on the operation site. This will put greater strain on the other bony prominences and great care must be taken to protect these. The wounds of the ischium and sacrum must be isolated from faecal material and the area kept dry so that it is often necessary to catheterise the patient. Most of the wounds will have drains inserted and suction drains are left in for several days until the drainage ceases. A record of the daily drainage is kept. The sutures are left in place for 12 to 14 days.

Physiotherapy

Pre-operative exercises are given to increase the circulation, prevent thrombosis, decrease oedema and prevent joint stiffness. Paraplegic patients may have flexion and adduction deformities, which need passive movement, but this is made more difficult by the presence of spasms. Postoperatively the physiotherapist will continue as necessary with passive movement of the joints and where possible will encourage active exercises but care must be taken not to disturb the grafts or flaps.

PILONIDAL SINUS

This is an abscess or sinus which forms in the natal cleft and contains hair and debris. Wide surgical excision eradicates the sinus but leaves a sizeable defect which either heals by epithelium growing from the edges with wound contraction, but this may take a long time, or it can be more speedily dealt with by skin grafting. The patient will be nursed on his front for some days. The patient can be encouraged to stay in this position by removing the head of the bed and turning the bed-head into the ward so that he then faces the centre of the ward and can see what is going on. As soon as the graft is stable, ambulation is commenced, but no sitting is allowed for 2 to 3 weeks. The patient is then instructed on keeping the area cleaned and bathed.

VARICOSE ULCERS

These develop usually in the lower leg in association with incompetence of the long and short saphenous systems. They are particularly difficult to deal with if they are associated with a previous deep vein thrombosis (post-phlebotic leg). Bed rest and elevation are important, but more so is the regular cleansing of the ulcer by the nursing staff using eusol, and then the application of eusol and paraffin as a wet dressing either on its own or over paraffin jelly gauze if the dressings become adherent. It is helpful for a dirty wound to be treated frequently, up to three times a day, but once the area is covered with granulation tissue and epithelialisation begins frequent dressings can be harmful as they strip off the new epithelium as it attempts to spread across the surface. Sometimes a surgical de-slough in the operating theatre under a general anaesthetic can speed the healing. Once granulation tissue has formed a split skin graft is applied and if there is a complete take of the skin graft the patient can be mobilised 2 weeks after the operation but must wear a firm elastic support. Some surgeons expose the skin graft. This will need to be rolled by the nurse every 2 hours to evacuate serum and any haematoma. The technique is to use a dental roll or cotton wool wound round a throat swab, then to press on the collection of fluid starting at a medial point and rolling the cotton wool in an outward direction until the fluid escapes from the edge of the wound (see Fig. 3/4, p. 39).

VAGINOPLASTY

A new vagina can be constructed where there is congenital absence or hypoplasia of the vagina. The gynaecologist and the plastic surgeon work together to create a cavity in front of the rectum and then a split skin graft is introduced mounted rear side out over a mould. Postoperatively the patient is confined to bed for 7 days and then examined under an anaesthetic. A vaginal mould is replaced and although it will be changed and cleansed daily it must be kept in place for 6 months as there is a great danger of the skin graft contracting and obliterating the space. Retention of the mould is difficult. Sexual intercourse can be commenced 6 weeks after surgery.

FACIAL PALSY

Paralysis of the facial nerve (VIIth cranial nerve) is rarely congenital and more commonly due to trauma. This trauma may be surgical from the removal of an acoustic neuroma or parotid tumour or occasionally the nerve fails to recover after a Bell's palsy.

Nerve repair or nerve grafts are successful in young people if performed before the facial muscles have had time to atrophy, which is usually about 1 to 2 years after the damage. Nerve transfers are used by some, for instance the hypoglossal nerve which normally supplies the muscles of the tongue can be transferred to the end of the non-functioning facial nerve and after some months of recovery the face will move instead of the half of the tongue on the side of the transfer.

New techniques of muscle graft are still being developed for cases where the muscles may have degenerated. In middle-aged and elderly patients static fascial slings are used, the fascia being taken from the thigh, which leaves a long and quite painful wound. Transfer of the temporalis and masseter muscles gives a more dynamic lift to the paralysed face. Patients with facial palsy are acutely aware of the severe deformity. They also suffer from epiphora, because the orbicularis oculi muscle is paralysed and they cannot close the eye, so there is danger of exposure and damage to the cornea. An urgent tarsorrhaphy is undertaken if the cornea is exposed while the patient is asleep. In this operation the margins of the eyelid are sutured together over part of their extent, usually the lateral half centimetre. Another complaint of these patients is that they tend to bite the lax cheek muscles.

After the operation there is considerable swelling and the patient is nursed sitting up. They also have difficulty in taking food and fluids and a feeding cup with a spout can be of great assistance.

CHAPTER THIRTEEN

The Role of the Social Worker and Resettlement

THE SOCIAL WORKER

The basic principle of the reorganised Health Service is that the patient should receive integrated and comprehensive care. There is, however, always a danger that the medical needs of the patient in hospital are cared for to the exclusion of his social needs.

Admission to hospital is a time of crisis, even if the medical condition is minor. It brings a change in routine, separation from the family and friends, as well as entry into an unfamiliar world with a degree of depersonalisation. The interruption of the normal daily routine enforces a time for reflection and reappraisal of the patient's lifestyle and relationships; feelings which have been avoided in the hurly-burly of life intrude and can lead to depression and regression; many issues that have been avoided have to be faced and patients need help to rebuild their lives. Even the patient who has had frequent admissions to hospital needs support as his tolerance begins to decrease. The value of a team approach is often not recognised or, perhaps, cannot be carried out because of limited resources: fortunately, burns and plastic surgery is one of the specialties where this concept is currently acknowledged and practised.

Essentially, the tasks of the social worker are non-scientific but in practice the range of work is wide. The treatment team must be aware of the contribution that a social worker can make so that full use can be made of her services; they must also realise that some patients resent such an intrusion and may refuse the help of the social worker.

The functions of the social worker are as follows:

1. To establish rapport with the patient, gaining his confidence to know his needs.
2. To enable the patient and relatives to come to terms with the illness.
3. To help the patient in obtaining benefits and improvement in home circumstances.
4. As a co-therapist, particularly in psychiatric disorders.

Early involvement of the social worker is important. If a patient with severe injuries is admitted the social worker might be able to be present to greet the relatives while the nursing staff are receiving the patient.

Burns patients

There is a far higher risk of a burn injury occurring to certain adults and children, for example members of the ethnic groups who are unused to the cold as well as British heating systems; deprived families in poor housing conditions; families with large numbers of children; the aged; the alcoholic and the drug abuser; certain pre-existing medical conditions, such as epilepsy or depressive illness. While the patient is in need of urgent medical treatment it is the waiting relatives who need the attention of the social worker. They usually want to talk about the incident, the events that surround it, the patient and their own feelings.

A burns unit accepts patients from a wide area. The relatives may have to travel a considerable distance to see the patients and they will have worries about children left hastily at home. In addition there may be financial concerns, particularly if it is the bread winner who is injured and he is self-employed. The parents of children admitted as patients feel guilty because they feel they have failed to protect the child. Quite often, relatives' anxiety may express itself not in tears but in anger. An experienced social worker can help to calm the situation, give encouragement and foster confidence in the treatment being administered. At the same time, much valuable information about the patient's background can be gained and the rapport established will form the basis for future work. While the patient is in a critical state the social worker's contact with him is brief but as treatment progresses so the focus of the social worker's attention will change from the relatives to the patient.

Obviously, practical problems, damaged accommodation, application for industrial injury benefit, care of dependants, even the booked holiday which will not be taken, need to be dealt with, and these loom large in the mind of the patient. But it is the psychological stresses which must be closely monitored. The patient is in an alien environment and has lost all the usual indicators that give him identity. His body looks different, often giving off an unpleasant smell; he is in an unfamiliar type of bed, embarrassingly short of clothing. His visitors may be strangely garbed in protective clothing and unable to touch him in an expression of affection or comfort. He has to undergo painful, frightening and prolonged procedures. The days seem interminable; his eyes may be injured so he cannot read, or his eyes may be uninjured but his hands bandaged so though he can see to read he cannot turn the pages. There is endless time to think, about the past, its joys and its disappointments, about the uncertainties of the future about the relationships with others. Will a wife want a man whose earning power has diminished? Will a husband want to caress a scarred body? Many patients will go through a period of regression which may take many forms.

The child with burns

The fear that all patients experience is heightened for the child. The majority of accidents take place at home and the child will feel that his safe little world has suddenly tumbled around his ears. He cannot be cuddled, held or patted to reassure him and no one can explain to him why this bond with his mother has been broken and other unfamiliar things are happening. This is particularly so for the really young children without language. The older child is frightened by the sight of his body and confinement to bed leads to frustration. This is demonstrated by behavioural changes. It is important that links with home are maintained and financial help may be necessary to assist the mother with regular visits. A family with a low income, or where the mother has to work, is worst hit. Those in receipt of supplementary benefits usually receive adequate help but there are no definite rules and only guidelines regarding the payment of travelling expenses. Some DHSS managers are less generous than others and the social worker will need to negotiate on behalf of the family and patient. When the child is admitted to hospital some of the supplementary allowance is lost and the social worker needs to have a knowledge of how and where a grant may be obtained. Unfortunately, grants are becoming fewer and the contributions made by the National Association for the Welfare of Children in Hospital are very welcome.

The mother's feeling of guilt when her child suffers injury may be exacerbated by criticism from relatives or neighbours. She often feels inadequate when she sees the expert handling of her child in hospital and may resent the control that the staff has over her child. She may well react by over-indulging the child or allowing her anxiety to communicate itself to her offspring. She can be encouraged to vent her feelings on the social worker rather than the child or other members of the family. It may be possible for her to link up with other mothers in similar situations, whose experience may be invaluable.

Non-accidental injury

When children are admitted with scalds and burns the possibility of non-accidental injury must be taken into account and the medical staff taking the history on admission will ask for detailed information about the incident – the time, place and who was present – so as to assess whether the circumstances match the injury. The social worker may also need to carry out checks on the family background before this possibility can be eliminated. There are procedures laid down which must be observed if there are grounds for suspicion. Even if there is no evidence of child abuse, very often there are stresses which may have lowered the level of protection: mother may be pregnant, a sibling ill, a relative may have died, or father may have lost his job.

Continuing care of the adult patient

The medical staff require a full social report on the patient as early as possible and it is useful to have the information easily available so that any problems can be discussed at each ward round. The information is needed when decisions on medical management, such as time of grafting or date of discharge from hospital, are made.

Much of this information is confidential and it is important that no unnecessary information is passed on.

Discharge from hospital

As the time approaches for the patient to leave hospital both he and his relatives need to be prepared. For many this is the beginning of a long period of adjustment to a changed situation. He will meet friends who are at a loss as to what to say and strangers who are upset by the appearance of the scarring. There may be disappointment because of the unrealistic expectation of what plastic surgery can achieve and the realisation that further admissions to hospital will be necessary. There may be anxiety at the thought of leaving a sheltered environment where there is skilled help. The patient may be returning to a stressful situation such as poor housing, emotional problems and so forth which were the cause of the accident.

Where a child is involved the local health visitor will have been contacted at the time of admission. She should now be informed of the discharge. The family may already be known to the local social worker. If not, the social services must be alerted and assistance such as home help, day care or continuing support requested. Many patients appreciate an opportunity to keep in touch with the hospital social worker, either when they attend outpatients or by a home visit. They will have confidence in the worker who knows and understands what they have been through in the initial injury and the subsequent treatment.

THE PLASTIC SURGERY UNIT

A large proportion of the patients admitted to the general wards of the unit will have psychological problems. Some patients will be disfigured causing lack of confidence and depression; they may be handicapped and unable to return to a job and the disability may cause problems with the relationships within the family and there is anxiety as to how a partner's feelings will change. The patient may suffer 'bereavement' through the loss of a limb or facial unsightliness and it is not uncommon for such patients to experience a grief reaction.

The parents of a baby with a congenital deformity may have feelings of failure or guilt, and the social worker can help by encouraging them to talk about these feelings. Occasionally, parents blame each other for what has happened and need to be together in order to explore their feelings openly with someone outside the family.

The social problems of plastic surgery patients can be considerable and all ages are involved. Many have a history of alcoholism, drug taking and psychological problems of all kinds; adults may have marital and relationship difficulties; some, both adults and children, may be in trouble with the law and be facing court proceedings. There are likely to be practical worries such as arranging transport, finances or accommodation, with which the social worker can help.

Another group of clients for the social worker are patients with malignant disease, some of whom may be dying. Advice and help will be needed for the relatives. There will also be a proportion of patients with incurable conditions who are chronically disabled, such as those with multiple sclerosis and paraplegia. For patients who are likely to have a temporary or permanent tracheostomy, the social worker should establish a relationship with the patient prior to surgery.

The social worker needs to be exceptionally alert to non-verbal communications from the patient and be able to respond to the mood of the moment. The patient's awareness can fluctuate so that one day he is able to accept the true situation while another day he will deny it. For those who do not want to know that they have malignant disease, care must be taken to respect this. Others welcome a social worker who can discuss the presence of a cancer and allow the patient to talk frankly about his feelings. It is important to maintain or strengthen the relationship between the patient and his relatives and to support the relatives at all times. Relatives need to be prepared for the eventual death of the patient. This is particularly hard when it is a child who has cancer.

The role of the social worker is one of liaison. In addition to communicating with outside agencies, there is liaison between patient and the medical and nursing staff. The patient often needs help in understanding the procedures planned for him, and by making the nursing and medical staff aware of the patient's social and emotional problems they have a better understanding of his behaviour. Open visiting, which is now standard on all children's wards, may cause problems between parents and nursing staff: the over-anxious parent who is aware of her child's needs can quickly cause irritation by constant demands; visitors who fail to appreciate that busy staff are impeded by delay in making it possible for them to carry out treatment; unruly siblings running up and down and waking sick children, quickly makes for a breakdown of goodwill. Nursing staff can become upset when they have to subject a child to unpleasant things such as distasteful medicines, uncomfortable injections and painful dressings while the parents give all the comforts. Having an easy relationship with all concerned enables the social worker to give support to both sides and calm the situation. Nursing staff too are people with backgrounds which may include problems; they work in highly charged atmospheres such as a burns unit and it is not surprising that they experience stress from time to time. They too may appreciate the support of the social worker and welcome her readiness to listen to their worries.

In summary, the social worker is an enabler; as a skilled listener she helps the patient to identify his problems and with support and information, to find his own solutions and make adjustments. She does this by spending time with the patient alone, with a relative, or, when the need arises, with the whole family. She encourages them to give vent to their anger, frustrations and fears in a controlled situation. The social worker is a liaiser between patient and medical and nursing staff and between the patient and the outside world. She is invited to take part in teaching activities from time to time and she also has a place in acting in a supportive role to other staff members. It is a demanding, exhausting and often saddening task she undertakes but, most would agree, extremely fascinating and certainly rewarding.

RESETTLEMENT

The early return to work of a wage earner is of paramount importance. This is frequently hindered by the patient's desire for a perfect result, the settlement of insurance claims and resistance from the employers. In the authors' unit a rehabilitation officer is employed by the hospital and is responsible for seeing that the patient returns to suitable employment as soon as possible after discharge from hospital. Usually, however, it is the medical staff and social workers who perform this function. They may obtain assistance from the disablement resettlement officer (DRO); unfortunately, he may only be able to begin work when the doctor considers the patient fully fit for employment. It is preferable that arrangements for return to work should be made while the patient is still recovering. Early return to work benefits the patient's recovery; this is particularly so in hand injuries as the activities of work or everyday use increases the mobility far faster than intermittent physiotherapy. There will be fewer difficulties with the employers and, contrary to popular belief, the value of compensation claims are not decreased by an early return to work. At the same time, a too early return, when the patient is unable to manage, can be demoralising and extremely harmful to recovery.

The person responsible for resettlement should ensure that he is informed within 48 hours of the admission of a wage earner suffering from an injury which could affect his return to work. This early referral has great advantages: the patient's anxiety about his job and wage-earning ability can be aired and his fears allayed. He is given a practical aim from the commencement of treatment thus reducing the chance of loss of morale, lack of motivation and poor co-operation with treatment.

Resettlement involves close co-ordination between the medical treatment team, industry and outside agencies such as the DRO. The *rehabilitation officer,* or social worker, will obtain advice from the hospital doctor, nursing staff, physiotherapist, occupational therapist and general practitioner to enable him to assess the patient's suitability for a particular job as well as his attitude towards work, and he will have to monitor the patient's progress towards recovery. A proportion of the time must be spent in the industrial environment, consulting management, workers on the shop floor and their representatives. He must have a practical knowledge of industry and industrial processes. A personal approach to employers at an early stage is helpful and often essential to the interests of the patient. It will be necessary for him to know precisely the type of job at which the patient was engaged, his experience in this job and his experience in other fields. It is useful to find out whether there is alternative employment in the same firm or whether a modification of the old job is possible to match the patient's particular disability. It may be possible to provide padded handles for machines where a patient's hands are scarred or have limited power grip. Alterations may have to be made providing wide doors and ramps for a wheelchair. A patient with severe facial disfigurement may need to be placed in a secluded working area and the working place of lower limb amputees should be on the ground floor if possible. Government grants are available to assist with the cost of alterations and firms will be more willing to co-operate if they are told of these facilities.

The patient will rarely return to work immediately after discharge from hospital and the burden of certification falls on the general practitioner. It is important, therefore, that the resettlement officer and the hospital doctor inform and liaise with the family doctor so that there are no errors in arranging the date for return to work. Some patients will manipulate a doctor to produce a certificate so that they remain off work.

The patient will need encouragement immediately he returns to work, particularly if the absence has been long. Early rising and the discipline of a daily routine appear irksome and daunting and a visit by the rehabilitation officer on his first day is of great value. Three months after return to work and at five years, the patients are reviewed by questionnaire. Problems are frequently encountered because of an alteration in the patient's condition which may have improved or deteriorated. The work available may have changed or the protected situation may be unacceptable to other employees or their representatives. Should these problems arise the rehabilitation officer should arrange a visit to the work-place and try to negotiate an acceptable solution.

Some patients are unable to return to their former employment and many jobs are incapable of modification without loss of efficiency or productivity. The building industry is particularly prone to these problems because of the heavy manual work, rough ground and the necessity to climb ladders and scaffolding. Under these circumstances some form of retraining has to be considered so that lighter employment can be undertaken.

Further Reading

The following is only a select list of books relating to plastic and reconstructive surgery. Most of these titles will have further lists and suggestions to allow the interested reader to delve more deeply into the subject.

Bernstein, N. (1976). *Emotional Care of the Facially Burned and Disfigured*. Little Brown and Co, Boston.

Cason, J. S. (1981). *Treatment of Burns*. Chapman and Hall, London.

Collyer, H. (1985). *Facial Disfigurement. Successful Rehabilitation*. Macmillan Press, London.

Conolly, W. B. (1980). *A Colour Atlas of Hand Conditions*. Wolfe Medical and Scientific Publications, London.

Davies, D. (1985). *An ABC of Plastic and Reconstructive Surgery*. BMA Publications, London.

Grabb, W. C. and Smith, J. W. (1973). *Plastic Surgery: A Concise Guide to Clinical Practice*. Little Brown and Co, Boston.

Harvey Kemble, J. V. and Lamb, B. E. (1984). *Plastic Surgical and Burns Nursing*. Ballière Tindall, Eastbourne.

Jackson, I. T. (ed.) (1981). *Recent Advances in Plastic Surgery 2*. Churchill Livingstone, Edinburgh.

McGregor, I. A. (1980). *Fundamental Techniques of Plastic Surgery and their Surgical Applications*, 7th edition. Churchill Livingstone, Edinburgh.

Muir, I. F. K. and Barclay, T. L. (1974). *Burns and their Treatment*. Lloyd Luke (Medical Books) Limited, London.

Piff, C. (1985). *Let's Face It*. Gollancz, London.

Wynn Parry, C. B. (1981). *Rehabilitation of the Hand*, 4th edition. Butterworths, London.

Useful Organisations

There are a number of self-help groups throughout the United Kingdom.

The Patients Association
Room 33, 18 Charing Cross Road
London WC2H OHR   01–240 0671

This association publishes a handbook *Self-Help and the Patient.*

Let's Face It
PO Box 4000, London W3 6XJ

Cleft Lip and Palate Association (CLAPA)
c/o Dental Department, Hospital for Sick Children
Great Ormond Street, London WC1N 3JH

The Mastectomy Association of Great Britain
26 Harrison Street, off Grays Inn Road
London WC1H 8JG

Society of Skin Camouflage and Disfigurement Therapy
Wester Pitmenzies, Auchtermuchty, Fife

McIndoe Burns Supporters
c/o Martin Bovey, 1 Delafield Road, London SE7 7NN

Cancer Care
c/o Margaret Hill
5 Courtney Drive, Emmer Green, Reading, Berks RG4 8XH

National Association for the Welfare of Children in Hospital
7 Exton Street, London SE1 8UE   01–261 1738

Index